T0353611

50^{PLUS}
Foot Challenges

*This book is dedicated
to Diane McMillan
and
Eilidh and Mhairi
Arran, Rory and Caitlin*

Publisher: Sarena Wolfaard
Development Editor: Nicola Lally
Project Manager: Elouise Ball
Designer/Design Direction: Charles Gray
Illustration Manager: Merlyn Harvey
Illustrator: Robert Britton

SECOND EDITION

50+

PLUS

Foot Challenges

Assessment and Evidence-Based Management

Colin E Thomson, PhD FCPod(S)
Senior Lecturer
Queen Margaret University, Edinburgh
Specialist Podiatrist, The Royal Infirmary of Edinburgh

J N Alastair Gibson, MD FRCS(orth)
Consultant Trauma and Orthopaedic Surgeon
The Royal Infirmary of Edinburgh; Part-time Senior Lecturer,
The University of Edinburgh

Foreword by

Malcolm Macnicol

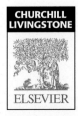

Edinburgh London New York Oxford Philadelphia St Louis Sydney Toronto 2009

CHURCHILL
LIVINGSTONE
ELSEVIER

An imprint of Elsevier Limited

First edition ©2002, Elsevier Limited. All rights reserved.
Second edition ©2009, Elsevier Limited. All rights reserved.

No part of this publication may be reproduced or transmitted in any form or by any means, electronic or mechanical, including photocopying, recording, or any information storage and retrieval system, without permission in writing from the publisher. Permissions may be sought directly from Elsevier's Rights Department: phone: (+1) 215 239 3804 (US) or (+44) 1865 843830 (UK); fax: (+44) 1865 853333; email: healthpermissions@elsevier.com. You may also complete your request online via the Elsevier website at www.elsevier.com/permissions.

ISBN 978-0-443-10402-2

British Library Cataloguing in Publication Data
A catalogue record for this book is available from the British Library

Library of Congress Cataloging in Publication Data
A catalog record for this book is available from the Library of Congress

Notice
Knowledge and best practice in this field are constantly changing. As new research and experience broaden our knowledge, changes in practice, treatment and drug therapy may become necessary or appropriate. Readers are advised to check the most current information provided (i) on procedures featured or (ii) by the manufacturer of each product to be administered, to verify the recommended dose or formula, the method and duration of administration, and contraindications. It is the responsibility of the practitioner, relying on their own experience and knowledge of the patient, to make diagnoses, to determine dosages and the best treatment for each individual patient, and to take all appropriate safety precautions. To the fullest extent of the law, neither the Publisher nor the Authors assume any liability for any injury and/or damage to persons or property arising out of or related to any use of the material contained in this book.

The Publisher

ELSEVIER
your source for books,
journals and multimedia
in the health sciences
www.elsevierhealth.com

Working together to grow
libraries in developing countries
www.elsevier.com | www.bookaid.org | www.sabre.org

ELSEVIER   BOOK AID International   Sabre Foundation

The
publisher's
policy is to use
**paper manufactured
from sustainable forests**

Printed in China

Contents

This book takes a novel approach to foot disorders. The two authors, one a podiatrist and the other an orthopaedic surgeon, guide us through the diagnosis and management of some common (and some not so common) disorders, using illustrated case histories. This practical approach is akin to taking part in a teaching session in the outpatient clinic, and is much more realistic than reading abstract descriptions in a textbook. Those learning about foot disorders for the first time will pick up a lot of valuable information, and more experienced practitioners will also find a great deal to interest them.

Foot disorders are responsible for a great deal of misery, and anything that helps to improve the diagnosis of common foot conditions and their correct treatment is to be welcomed. I enjoyed reading this book and I am sure that you will too.

Geoffrey Hooper MMSc FRCS FRCSEd (orth)

The normal foot offers propulsion, support and sensitivity to the most subtle of forces and stimuli. Yet it is often ignored in clinical practice and the consequences of its disorder can be dire. The realisation that podiatric problems are worthy of specialised attention has led to a recent and rapid expansion both in the clinical services and the number of trained practitioners versed in the relevant anatomy, physiology and pathological processes of the foot – a welcome trend.

Colin Thomson and Alastair Gibson have combined most successfully in producing a comprehensive vade mecum which meets this burgeoning interest. The first edition described medical and surgical conditions, including congenital and acquired foot disorders in childhood. The vivid colour portrayal of a wide variety of foot problems encountered in the surgery or clinic once again characterises this second edition, while the accompanying text is succinct, practically orientated and supported by reference to the relevant literature. Importantly, a section is devoted to 'the foot at risk' while potentially dangerous surgical interventions have been submitted to cautious appraisal.

It is a pleasure to welcome this revised and enlarged second edition. For the inexperienced and the experienced alike this compact book will offer much of interest, couched within a thorough and sensible approach to the afflictions of the foot.

M F Macnicol BSc(hons) MCh FRCS FRCP FRCSEd(orth)
Dip Sports Med

In compiling this book, it has been our aim to provide a self-assessment text that allows the reader to test their knowledge on a wide variety of conditions of the foot, some common, some less so. It has not been our ambition to design a comprehensive reference text on the foot; for this purpose there are already many excellent texts available. Instead we have tried to make available useful information in a concise and accessible format that is easy to read and user friendly, with a prominent pictorial content.

We offer you 50 cases designed to present a series of challenges to all those involved in treating the foot. We have set the reader problems of varying difficulty, the solutions for which are suggested overleaf with an expanded discussion of the condition in question. Key references are listed as well as summary points. We have included, where appropriate, 'clinical tips' which will aid your practice.

It is not essential to use this book as a self-assessment text, as it will serve equally well as a short guide to a broad range of foot conditions. For your convenience we have grouped these into seven sections.

We hope that by the end of this text you will have graduated to become a 'foot expert'.

During the last decade there has been an increasing realization that clinical practice should be based on sound scientific evidence. In this edition we have attempted to bring evidence to the fore where and when it exists. This, we hope, will allow the reader to synthesize the available data, reference any meta-analyses and make rational management decisions. We also recognize that knowledge should be underwritten by some form of assessment. To this end we have introduced an MCQ section at the end of the book covering a selection of material from the text. The questions are formatted as single best answer.

We have retained the layout that was popular in the first edition but revamped the book, adding three new sections: sports injuries, 'lumps and bumps' and a plenary section incorporating the multiple choice questions. There are over 100 additional illustrations and completely updated references. In all, 15 new challenges are presented that we hope the reader will find stimulating. These range from a condition presenting primarily in the tropics to one commonly afflicting athletes. Complete the challenges and we hope you will have a sound base for your practice.

Acknowledgements

We are indebted to Mr Mike Devlin, Steve Stanton and Frances Gilles of the Department of Clinical Photography at the Royal Infirmary of Edinburgh who expertly took most of the clinical photographs printed in this book. We also thank Judith Watson for her drawings and Malcolm Macnicol (Figs 1.1–1.6) and Donald Salter (Figs 11.3 and 44.3) for providing clinical slides. Figure 22.1 was kindly supplied by Professor Steffen Breusch, Consultant Orthopaedic Surgeon, Royal Infirmary, Edinburgh, Figure 34.1 by Dimension Photography, Sharnford, UK, Figure 34.2 by Derek Locke (www.geocities.com/braguk), Figure 34.3 by Michael Dye (www.floridaback@yardsnakes.com) and Figure 52.1 by Mr Tim Theologis, Consultant Orthopaedic Surgeon, Nuffield Orthopaedic Centre, Oxford.

Abbreviations

ABPI	Ankle brachial pressure index
BJHS	Benign joint hypermobility syndrome
CRP	C-reactive protein
DEXA	Dual energy X-ray absorptiometry
ESR	Erythrocyte sedimentation rate
ESWT	Extracorporeal shock wave therapy
FDL	Flexor digitorum longus
GCTTS	Giant cell tumour of the tendon sheath
HPV	Human papilloma virus
IP	Interphalangeal
MTP	Metatarsophalangeal

MRI	Magnetic resonance imaging
MRSA	Methicillin-resistant *Staphylococcus aureus*
PTT	Posterior tibial tendon
PVNS	Pigmented villonodular synovitis
PUVA	Psoralen ultraviolet light (band A)
RCT	Randomized controlled trial
SACH	Solid ankle cushion heel
UVA	Ultraviolet light (band A)

Section 1

Paediatrics

Case 1

A young woman gives birth in midsummer to a daughter. It is immediately evident that the child has severe deformities of both feet (Fig. 1.1).

1. What is the approximate incidence and likely aetiology of this condition?
2. What are the characteristic radiological appearances?
3. What would be appropriate initial treatment?
4. At what stage would surgery be contemplated?

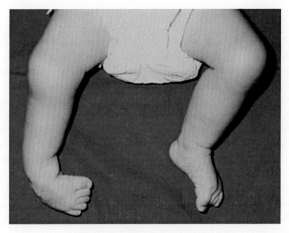

Fig. 1.1 Bilateral foot deformities

Congenital talipes equinovarus

1. Clubfoot has an incidence of approximately 1 in 1000 live births. In the majority the condition is labelled as 'idiopathic', although the deformity is associated with myelomeningocele, amniotic band syndrome (Streeter's dysplasia) and arthrogryposis. Population and twin studies suggest a genetic component but the mode of inheritance does not follow a distinctive pattern. In the presence of a gene mutation, such as polymorphism in the methylenetetrahydrofolate reductase gene (MTHFR), other factors will predispose the child to contraction of the soft tissues of the foot and abnormal talar development. Deformity is exacerbated by a reduction in maternal amniotic fluid (oligohydramnios), hence the prevalence of the condition in children born during the summer months, and by disturbances in neuromuscular function producing ipsilateral calf muscle hypoplasia.

2. The primary deformities are those of hindfoot equinus and varus with forefoot adductus and supination. This positioning is secondary to medial and plantar deviation of the talar neck, medial rotation of the calcaneus and medial displacement of the navicular and cuboid. This leads to a parallel and superimposed positioning of the talus upon the calcaneus (angle <20°) and a negative talus/first metatarsal angle as shown in Figure 1.2a and b. On a dorsiflexion lateral film the talocalcaneal angle is reduced (< normal 35°; Fig. 1.2c and d).

3. A gradual improvement in anatomical alignment is achieved by sequential stretching. The key, according to Ponseti, is a reversal of the cavus by dorsiflexion of the first metatarsal during the initial stage of treatment. Supination and equinus are accepted until the metatarsal is adequately dorsiflexed. Reduction in the cavus unlocks the midfoot. Subsequent correction occurs by using the uncovered talar head as a lateral fulcrum. As the forefoot is then abducted, the heel externally rotates and dorsiflexes, reversing the equinus. The position is held by applying a dynamic splint, as shown in Figure 1.3, or plaster casts applied with the knee in at least 70° of flexion. It is necessary for the physician or a trained therapist to see the child weekly to ensure that the splintage is holding the foot in the corrected position. After 2 or 3 months, if an adequate correction has been achieved, the feet may be splinted out with an abduction bar attached to the shoes. This will be used full time for 3 months and then required as a night splint to age 3 or 4 (Fig. 1.4).

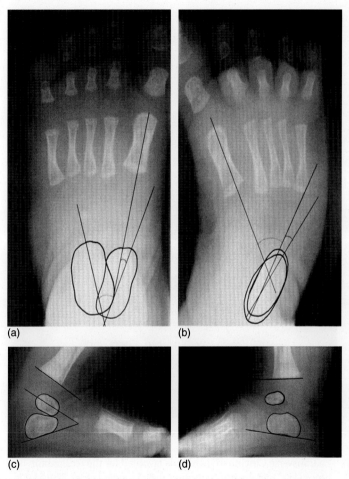

Fig. 1.2 Radiography of club foot: normal alignment (a) compared with parallelism of talus and calcaneus (b). Lateral radiography: normal (c) compared with parallelism on stress dorsiflexion (d)

4. The optimal timing of surgery and the exact procedures required remain a matter of some debate. The majority of surgeons would probably agree that at least a lengthening of the Achilles tendon should be considered after 3 months if conservative measures fail. In Edinburgh, an extended posteromedial release through

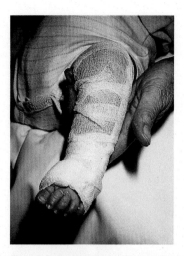

Fig. 1.3 Dynamic splintage with strapping

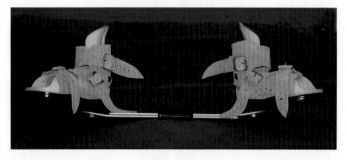

Fig. 1.4 Ponseti ankle foot orthosis abduction brace (www.c-prodirect.co.uk)

a transverse Cincinnati incision is favoured for the recalcitrant foot (Fig. 1.5), creating a mobile and plantigrade foot. The foot is immobilized in plaster following surgery to maintain the corrected position. The success of surgery relates to the compliance with bracing. Studies from the Ponseti Clubfoot Center in New York suggest that two-thirds of those non-compliant with bracing had recurrence of deformity, with one-third of these requiring more extensive surgery than Achilles tenotomy and anterior tibial tendon transfer. In contrast, only 14% of those compliant with bracing had recurrences and none required extensive surgery.

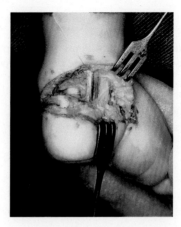

Fig. 1.5 Extended posteromedial release

Key points

- Clubfoot is the most common orthopaedic deformity at birth and requires careful early management.
- Splinting, augmented by a percutaneous Achilles tendon release, will suffice in many instances.
- Surgical intervention should be considered after 3 months if conservative measures fail.

Further reading

Abdelgawad AA, Lehman WB, van Bosse HJ, Scher DM, Sala DA (2007) Treatment of idiopathic clubfoot using the Ponseti method: minimum 2-year follow-up. Journal of Pediatric Orthopedics 16(2):98–105.

Dobbs MT, Nunley R, Schoenecker PL (2006) Long-term follow-up of patients with clubfeet treated with extensive soft-tissue release. Journal of Bone and Joint Surgery 88-A:986–96.

Macnicol MF (2003) The management of club foot: issues for debate. Journal of Bone and Joint Surgery 85-B:167–70.

Macnicol MF, Nadeem RD (2000) Evaluation of the deformity in club foot by somatosensory evoked potentials. Journal of Bone and Joint Surgery 82-B:731–5.

Ponseti IV, Zhivkov M, Davis N, Sinclair M, Dobbs MB, Morcuende JA (2006) Treatment of the complex idiopathic clubfoot. Clinical Orthopaedics and Related Research 451:171–6.

Case 2

A girl is having increasing pain when standing for prolonged periods. She is aware of tender 'lumps' in her insteps as shown in Figure 2.1.

1. What is causing this swelling?
2. What condition is it associated with?
3. Is surgical resection feasible?

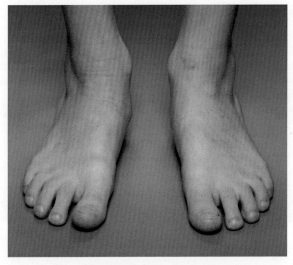

Fig. 2.1 Medial prominences on the side of the feet

Accessory navicular

1. This patient presents with an accessory navicular ossicle (os tibiale externum). It usually lies posteromedial to the navicular tuberosity and will almost always receive at least a part of the tibialis posterior insertion. Usually there is a small joint between the main bone and the developmental ossicle, but in some instances there is a fibrous bridge. In effect, there are two types:
   - Type 1 is a small sesamoid bone within the tendon itself, anatomically separate from the navicular
   - Type 2 (Fig. 2.2) is a bone developed from a separate ossification centre within the main cartilage mass of the navicular itself.

2. Patients may suffer from mild flatfoot as evident in Figure 2.1. This is rarely sufficient to prevent the patient rising onto single leg tip-toe.

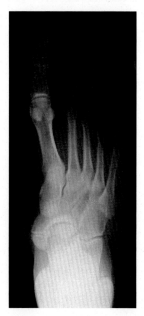

Fig. 2.2 Large accessory navicular

3. Approximately 5% of the population have an accessory navicular and most manage well. In a few patients surgery is required. This is usually due to inflammation of an overlying bursa or to pain arising secondary to chondromalacia of the intervening joint. In many cases the ossicle may be excised by a direct approach, leaving the tibialis posterior tendon intact. If this is not possible then the main insertion of the tendon must be rerouted. The tendon is taken off from the accessory with a small flake of bone. After excising the remainder of the ossicle, the tendon is then reattached onto the plantar surface of the main bone by a through-bone suture or use of a suture anchor.

Key points

- The accessory navicular is a normal anatomical variant.
- 99m-Technetium bone scanning may be helpful if the significance of the accessory bone is uncertain.
- Excision of the ossicle may be necessary.

Further reading

Kopp FJ, Marcus RE (2004) Clinical outcomes of surgical treatment of the symptomatic accessory navicular. Foot and Ankle International 25:27–30.

Macnicol MF, Voutsinas S (1984) Surgical treatment of the symptomatic accessory navicular. Journal of Bone and Joint Surgery 66:218–26.

Nakayama S, Sugimoto K, Takakura Y et al (2005) Percutaneous drilling of symptomatic accessory navicular in young athletes. American Journal of Sports Medicine 33:531–5.

Case 3

This girl's mother is concerned about her daughter's flat feet (Fig. 3.1a, b). She reports that her shoes develop an abnormal bulging on the medial side of the upper. There are no other symptoms and 'her feet have always been this way'. The heel rise test is shown in Figure 3.2.

1. Describe the clinical features seen in Figure 3.1. What do these features indicate?
2. What is the heel rise test (Fig. 3.2), which mechanism is it testing and what does it reveal?
3. What conditions are associated with flat foot in childhood?
4. Why is this parent concerned that her daughter has flat feet?

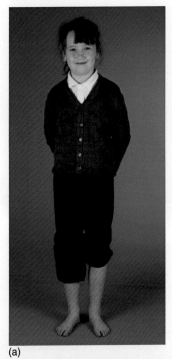

(a)

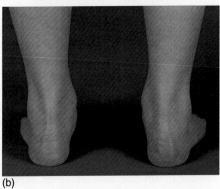

(b)

Fig. 3.1 Flat feet. (a) Standing view. (b) Posterior view

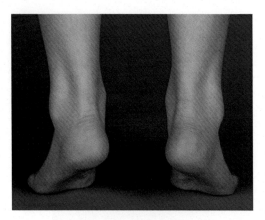

Fig. 3.2 Heel rise test

Flat foot

1. Flat foot (pes planus) is simply a low medial arch. In addition to this, the rearfoot is in a valgus alignment. In Figure 3.1 there is also evidence of Helbing's sign (bowing of the Achilles tendon), prominence of the medial malleolus and abduction of the forefoot. The combination produces pes planovalgus.
2. For the heel rise test, patients are asked to stand on their toes. Normally this will cause the medial longitudinal arch of the foot to increase in height and the calcaneus to invert (see Fig. 7.2). With rigidity, on toe standing the arch will fail to rise and there will be no inversion of the calcaneus. This test uses Hicks' windlass mechanism whereby dorsiflexion of the toes creates tension in the plantar fascia, drawing the forefoot and hindfoot closer. In so doing, this increases the arch and inverts the subtalar joint. An alternative to the heel rise test is Jack's test whereby, on standing, the patient's great toe is dorsiflexed at the MTP joint (Fig. 3.3). This should produce a similar effect to that described above. In this case, arch formation indicated that the flat foot was flexible, excluding a pathological condition such as tarsal coalition from the diagnosis (Chapter 7).

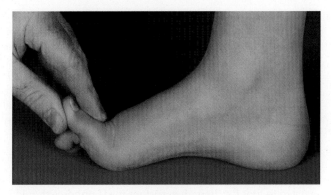

Fig. 3.3 Jack's test

3. Flat foot is associated with connective tissue disorders such as benign joint hypermobility syndrome, Marfan's and Ehlers–Danlos syndromes. Neuromuscular conditions such as cerebral palsy and poliomyelitis, rupture of the tibialis posterior tendon and juvenile chronic arthritis may also cause lowering of the medial longitudinal arch. Congenital causes are tarsal synostosis and congenital vertical talus. The latter produces a rare but very deforming example of flat foot (Fig. 3.4).

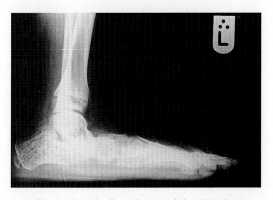

Fig. 3.4 Lateral radiograph: congenital vertical talus

4. Flat feet cause concern for parents because there is a perception that they are associated with pain in adulthood. The infant's foot is flat due to a plantar pad of fat and joint laxity. This lasts for about 1–2 years and then the medial longitudinal arch usually increases in height during childhood. Approximately 15% of adults have flat feet, low arches are seen in some races and foot shape is inherited to some extent. Bilateral flat foot in children and adolescents is usually asymptomatic and should not restrict sporting activities. It will not always cause disability during adulthood.

5. A painless flexible flat foot does not warrant surgical intervention. Reassurance should be given to the child and parent that it is a normal variant. If there is pain and it is related to foot function, then custom-made orthoses should be provided to hold the rearfoot in more neutral alignment and restore stability (Fig. 3.5). However, there is a lack of evidence to suggest that orthoses effect a permanent correction of the deformity, although they can improve foot function.

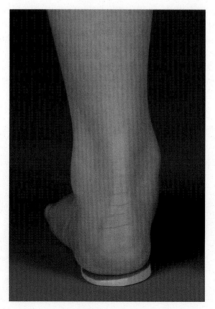

Fig. 3.5 Control of hindfoot position with medial wedging

Key points

- The heel rise test differentiates between a rigid and flexible flat foot.
- Flexible flat foot in children is common and is often a cause of parental concern. It does not usually require treatment.
- Custom-made orthoses should be considered on an individual basis.
- Surgery is never indicated and parents should be reassured.

Further reading

Harris EJ, Vanore JV, Thomas JL et al (2004) Clinical practice guideline pediatric flatfoot panel of the American College of Foot and Ankle Surgeons. Journal of Foot and Ankle Surgery 43(6):341–73.

Kitaoka HB, Lou ZP, An KN (1998) Three dimensional analysis of flat foot deformity: cadaver study. Foot and Ankle International 19(7):447–50.

Staheli LT (1999) Planovalgus foot deformity. Journal of the American Podiatric Medical Association 89:94–9.

Case 4

One of the most common presenting foot abnormalities in children is shown in Figure 4.1.

1. This common digital anomaly is universally described as what? How should management be approached? Is there ever any indication for surgery?

2. How does an overriding toe, as shown in Figure 4.2, differ in aetiology? Which eponym is commonly associated with the correction of this deformity and will surgery be successful?

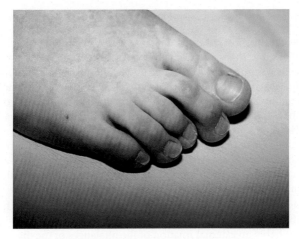

Fig. 4.1 Lesser digit deformity in a 14-year-old boy

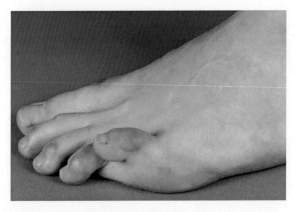

Fig. 4.2 Overriding fifth toe

Claw toe and adductus quinti digiti

1. By far the most common digital anomaly in children is the 'claw' toe. This arises from an imbalance between flexor and extensor muscle power and/or lumbrical muscle weakness. In the absence of a neurological deficit leading to clear evidence of leg muscle weakness, it may be worthwhile attempting to correct the toe clawing by asking the child to perform regular exercises. However, often these are of little value and more definitive surgery is required. The classic operation is that described by Girdlestone (see Taylor 1951), in which the flexor tendons are detached from the phalanges of the digit and transferred laterally and dorsally to be attached to the extensor tendon.

2. Adductus digiti quinti, or congenital contracture of the fifth toe, is generally a familial deformity. The initial deformity is probably an external rotation of the phalanges of the digit, causing change in the vector of action of the dorsal extensor tendon. The fifth toe is pulled dorsally over the fourth digit and with time the dorsal capsule of the MTP joint contracts.

   A variety of surgical procedures have been described to correct this deformity. These range from taking the distal end of the long extensor tendon and passing it under the digit from medial to lateral, as described by Lapidus in 1942, to resection of the base of the proximal phalanx and creation of a syndactyly between the fourth and fifth toes. The most common procedure is probably that termed Butler's operation, as shown in Figure 4.3. The authors'

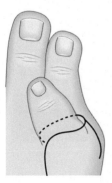 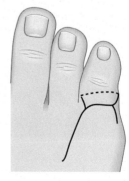

Fig. 4.3 Butler's operation

experience has been that this procedure is fine for young children but it seldom holds the toe in older subjects. Usually an osteotomy of the fifth metatarsal will be required to derotate the toe.

Key points

- Claw toes are generally familial and bilateral.
- Surgery may be required but should be performed before the age of 15 years.
- Overriding of the fifth toe is not easily corrected. The toe often looks short, especially if part of the proximal phalanx is resected.
- Long-term outcomes are not especially good and the patient should be warned that further surgery may be necessary.

Further reading

Cockin J (1968) Butler's operation for an overriding fifth toe. Journal of Bone and Joint Surgery 50-B:78–81.

Coughlin MJ (2002) Lesser toe abnormalities. Journal of Bone and Joint Surgery 84-A:1446–69.

Taylor RG (1951) The treatment of claw toes by multiple transfers of the flexor into extensor tendons. Journal of Bone and Joint Surgery 33:539–42.

Case 5

A 7-year-old boy presents with a 3-week history of right foot pain. He does not recall suffering any trauma. He is, however, noted to have a limp, offloading that foot, and examination reveals an area of tenderness to palpation along his medial longitudinal arch. The boy's left foot appears normal.

X-rays were requested and the images are shown in Figure 5.1.

1. What is this condition and who described it?
2. What is the aetiology?
3. How should the boy be treated?
4. Can the condition occur in adults?

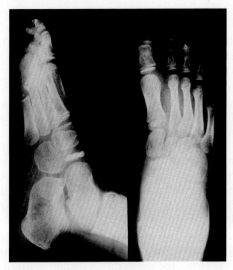

Fig. 5.1 Navicular collapse

Kohler's disease

1. The radiograph shows avascularity of the tarsal navicular. It was described in 1908 by the German physician Alban Kohler (1874–1947).

2. The precise aetiology is unknown but several hypotheses have been put forward based on the radiographic findings of bone flattening and sclerosis. Waugh examined the vascular pattern of the navicular, reporting his results in 1958. He found that most 5 year olds had an ossific nucleus that is supplied by five or six arteries although development of the bone is based on one of these. It was at an early stage, in the presence of a single vessel only, that he hypothesized that disruption of the blood supply would lead to ischaemia and fragmentation of the navicular.

3. Treatment is generally conservative with or without casting. Although the navicular at presentation will be flattened with irregular sclerosis, the appearances generally revert to normal within approximately 12 months. In the early phase of disease, bone scans may demonstrate decreased tracer uptake (photopenic region) but subsequently a hot area is identified due to the increased vascularity associated with 'repair'. In most reported series with long-term follow-up, virtually all patients are reported to be asymptomatic.

4. Adult-onset navicular osteonecrosis (Müller–Weiss or Brailsford's disease) most frequently presents in patients aged 40–50 years. Pes planovarus is typical due to the orientation of the talar head laterally. Treatment is by a localized fusion between the talus and navicular with or without incorporation of the cuneiforms into the fusion mass.

Key points

- Kohler's disease is probably an avascular necrosis of bone.
- Usually the condition is self-limiting in children.
- Pes planovarus characterizes the adult type.

Further reading

DiGiovanni CW, Patel A, Calfee R, Nickisch F (2007) Osteonecrosis in the foot. Journal of the American Academy of Orthopedic Surgeons 15:208–17.

Waugh W (1958) The ossification and vascularization of the tarsal navicular and their relation to Kohler's disease. Journal of Bone and Joint Surgery 40-B:765–77.

Williams GA, Cowell HR (1981) Kohler's disease of the tarsal navicular. Clinical Orthopaedics and Related Research 158:53–8.

Case 6

A 9-month-old child was brought by a very concerned mother to the paediatric clinic. Examination of the child's feet revealed a significant deformity (Fig. 6.1).

1. This deformity is fairly common. What is the primary abnormality and with what other conditions is it associated?
2. Would any form of conservative treatment be appropriate?
3. When will surgery become necessary and what operations have been described?
4. Is a good long-term outcome expected?

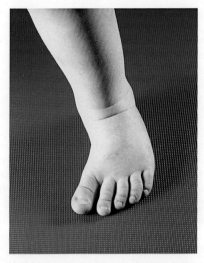

Fig. 6.1 Severe in-toeing in a child of 9 months

Metatarsus adductus

1. The illustration shows metatarsus adductus. In milder forms the soft tissues remain lax and it is generally possible to hold the foot in neutral alignment. In this case virtually no abduction was possible.

   The deformity in this instance occurred as an isolated deformity, but metatarsus adductus may be associated with clubfoot and developmental dysplasia of the hip.

2. Advice was sought from a paediatric orthopaedic surgeon and it was recommended that the deformity would correct with time. During the next few months the child was seen regularly by a physiotherapist who progressively stretched out the soft tissues.

3. Forefoot adduction may occur in patients with clubfoot (Chapter 1) if the midfoot becomes fixed and rigid or if the tibialis anterior muscle is relatively overactive.

   The simplest surgical procedure is probably to release the abductor hallucis tendon at the level of the first metatarsal neck, but this procedure is only of value in terms of reducing the duration of conservative therapy. Muscle imbalance must be directly addressed by either split or complete transfer of the tibialis anterior tendon laterally. In the more rigid foot, particularly in older children, a capsular release to mobilize the tarsometatarsal and intermetatarsal joints will be required or even osteotomies of the metatarsal bases to bring them round into correct alignment.

4. Outcomes from conservative treatment are generally excellent with minimal residual deformity. In this case the child had an entirely normal foot by age 3 years.

Key points

- Metatarsus adductus may be associated with clubfoot.
- Serial stretching and casting will generally allow remodelling to occur.

Further reading

Berman A, Gartland JJ (1971) Metatarsal osteotomy for the correction of adduction of the fore part of the foot in children. Journal of Bone and Joint Surgery 53-A:498–506.

Heyman CH, Herndon CH, Strong JM (1958) Mobilization of the tarsometatarsal and intermetatarsal joints for the correction of resistant adduction of the fore part of the foot in congenital club-foot or congenital metatarsus varus. Journal of Bone and Joint Surgery 40-A:299–310.

Wan SC (2006) Metatarsus adductus and skewfoot deformity. Clinical Podiatry Medicine and Surgery 23:23–40.

Case 7

This young man first presented for treatment of a painful flat left foot aged 12 years. He was offered no treatment at this time. However, he is now 17 and his pain has become progressively worse over the past few years. He is unable to play tennis and has chosen a sedentary job to avoid weightbearing. Examination reveals hindfoot valgus and flat foot (Fig. 7.1a, b), and the heel rise test is abnormal on the left side (Fig. 7.2).

1. Diagnose this young man's foot complaint.
2. Which pathognomonic radiological feature is apparent in Figure 7.3 and why does it occur with this condition?
3. Are there any further investigations you would consider?
4. List the treatment options.

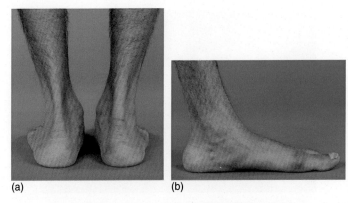

Fig. 7.1 (a) Posterior view of both feet. (b) Medial view of left foot

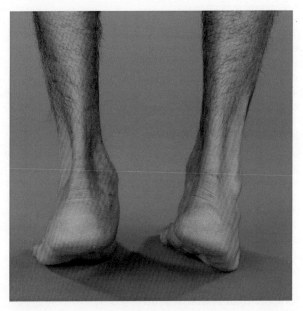

Fig. 7.2 Heel rise test: right hind heel inverts (normal), left hind foot remains in valgus (abnormal)

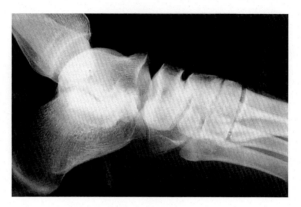

Fig. 7.3 Lateral radiograph of left foot

Talocalcaneal synostosis

1. Talocalcaneal synostosis (peroneal spastic flat foot, tarsal coalition) represents 48% of all tarsal synostoses. Coalition is usually of the medial facet (sustentaculum tali) but involvement of the posterior facet has also been reported. The condition becomes painful in the second decade as the cartilaginous bar ossifies. Examination reveals a loss of subtalar joint movement. Standing on tip toes will not correct the hindfoot valgus and therefore presents as a rigid flat foot (see Fig. 7.2).

2. X-rays are of limited value although flattening ('beaking') of the head of the talus is pathognomonic and results from abnormal demands on the talonavicular joint for frontal plane motion. The lack of subtalar and midtarsal motion will be countered by increased movement distally at the cuneiform metatarsal joints. These are therefore at risk from degenerative arthritis and will be a source of pain.

3. Harris views (ski-jump) projections demonstrate the subtalar joint, but CT scans are probably easier to interpret (Fig. 7.4). In this case radio-isotope bone scans were also taken that revealed hot spots in the midtarsal joints (Fig. 7.5).

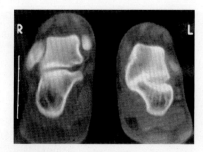

Fig. 7.4 CT image of subtalar joints showing union of the talus and calcaneus at the middle facet of the left sustentaculum talus

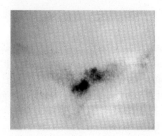

Fig. 7.5 Radio-isotope bone scan showing hot spot in midtarsal joint

4. Although footwear modifications such as medial arch supports may be helpful, conservative management is not always rewarding. In patients under about 14 years of age, where there are no degenerative changes, bar excision will diminish symptoms and lessen secondary arthritis. It is also possible to insert an implant into the subtalar joint to restore normal joint alignment. This patient presented too late for this treatment. Although a triple arthrodesis may be successful in the short term, cuneiform-metatarsal arthritis will follow as evident in radiographs taken from an older patient shown in Figure 7.6.

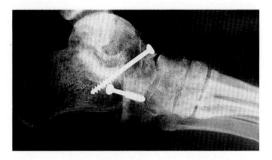

Fig. 7.6 Triple arthrodesis of left foot

Key points

- Talocalcaneal synostosis presents with a painful flat foot in children and young adults.
- The heel rise test differentiates between a rigid and flexible flat foot.
- 'Beaking' of the talus, apparent on lateral radiographs, is pathognomonic of the condition.
- CT imaging will delineate the extent of tarsal union.
- Early bar excision is recommended.

Further reading

Giannini S, Ceccarelli F, Vannini F, Baldi E (2003) Operative treatment of flatfoot with talocalcaneal coalition. Clinical Orthopaedics and Related Research 411:178–87.

Mann RA, Beaman DN, Horton G (1998) Isolated subtalar arthrodesis. Foot and Ankle International 19:511–19.

Varner KE, Michelson JD (2000) Tarsal coalition in adults. Foot and Ankle International 21:669–72.

Case 8

These two pictures show very different feet (Figs 8.1, 8.2).

1. What is the descriptive term used to describe the anomaly shown in Figure 8.1?
2. What are the other characteristics of this familial syndrome?
3. Name the term used to describe shortening of the metatarsals as shown in Figure 8.2.
4. Which metatarsals are most commonly affected and is surgery ever appropriate?

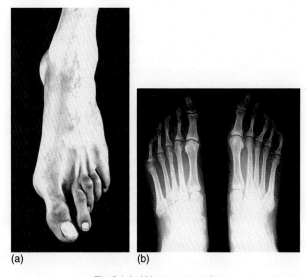

Fig. 8.1 (a, b) Long metatarsals

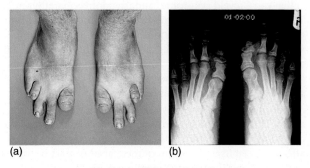

Fig. 8.2 (a, b) Short metatarsals

Congenital metatarsal anomalies

1. Figure 8.1 shows the foot of a patient with arachnodactyly (spider digits) and is virtually pathognomonic of Marfan's syndrome. This condition arises because of a mutation in the *FBN* 1 gene encoding fibrillin 1. It is transmitted as an autosomal dominant trait.

2. The condition is characterized by body disproportion with long limbs, dislocation of the lens, scoliosis, herniae and, in later life, aortic aneurysm. Most of these anomalies are attributable at least in part to ligamentous laxity, as fundamentally the disorder is a collagen disease. Pes planovalgus is present in approximately 25% of patients. The talus is usually tilted vertically.

   Arachnodactyly also occurs in another autosomal dominant condition known as congenital contractural arachnodactyly. Although there is a similar disproportionate body development as in Marfan's syndrome, the other features noted do not develop. Joint contracture is present from birth.

3. Shortening of the metatarsals is termed brachymetatarsia (brachymetapody). The patient shown in Figure 8.2 was suffering from spondyloepiphyseal dysplasia tarda, but the condition is also found in several other skeletal dysplasias, for example achondroplasia, chondroectodermal dysplasia (Ellis–van Creveld syndrome) and pseudohypoparathyroidism. These conditions are frequently autosomal dominant although they may arise as new mutations. Resection of 1.5 cm of the second and third metatarsal shafts, greatly improved the man's appearance (Fig. 8.3a, b). It was felt that lengthening of the short metatarsals would have been a significant undertaking for someone who was entirely asymptomatic.

4. A short fourth ray alone may also occur, as shown in Figure 8.4a and b. This condition is common in Japanese people and is caused by the premature closure of the epiphyseal plate of the affected metatarsal. The point of metatarsal contact is displaced proximally and the toe offloaded (Fig. 8.5).

   Treatment can be quite difficult. A one-stage lengthening with bone graft is rapid and economical because no external fixator is required. However, there are limitations to the length

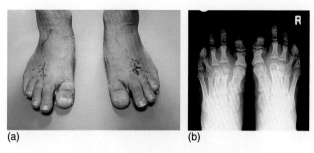

Fig. 8.3 (a, b) Post shortening metatarsal

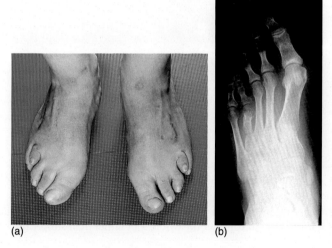

Fig. 8.4 (a, b) Congenitally short fourth ray post lengthening

that may be achieved, and complications such as MTP joint subluxation, necrosis of the toe due to vascular insufficiency and a potential for recurrence of shortening due to graft resorption are common. For these reasons distraction callotasis after metatarsal shaft osteotomy is probably now more popular.

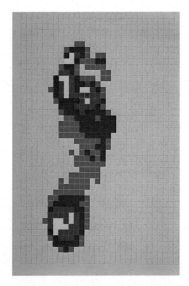

Fig. 8.5 Altered in-shoe contact pressure distribution (Musgrave® system)

Key points

- A congenital foot deformity is usually part of a generalized syndrome.
- Operative intervention will alter the biomechanics of the foot and it is essential to consider the whole foot rather than simply the deformed part.
- Metatarsal lengthening is limited by the resistance and length of associated neurovascular structures.

Further reading

Lindsey JM, Michelson JD, MacWilliams BA, Sponseller PD, Miller NH (1998) The foot in Marfan syndrome: clinical findings and weight-distribution patterns. Journal of Pediatric Orthopedics 18:755–9.

Shim JS, Park SJ (2006) Treatment of brachymetatarsia by distraction osteogenesis. Journal of Pediatric Orthopedics 26:250–4.

Lumps and bumps

Case 9

The lump on the dorsum of this middle-aged man's foot causes him pain when he is wearing shoes (Fig. 9.1a, b). He wonders if he can have the lump removed.

1. What is the aetiology of this condition?
2. Why do the radiographs not reflect the true situation?
3. What treatment is appropriate?

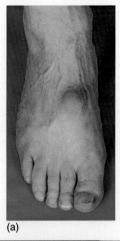

(a)

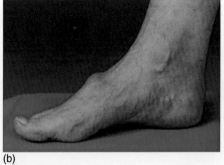

(b)

Fig. 9.1 (a) Dorsal and (b) lateral views of midfoot

Tarsometatarsal arthritis (tarsal boss)

1. The condition is associated with a hypermobile, plantarflexed first metatarsal. Repetitive impaction of the base of the first metatarsal against the medial cuneiform eventually has led to joint degeneration. There will be some erosion of the adjoining cartilage surfaces and an osteophytic ridge has formed on the joint margin. Pressure against the man's shoe has then caused skin irritation and the formation of a painful bursitis.

2. The lesion is often clinically much larger than the radiographic appearance. This is due to the presence of a cartilage cap covering the bony prominence that is not evident on X-ray (Fig. 9.2).

3. Unless the condition is especially troublesome, patients are usually advised against surgery. There is a high risk of recurrence and the surgical scar may be tender where it catches any footwear. Surgical removal of only the soft tissue swelling is futile as it does not address the underlying problem. It is important to 'saucerize' the underlying bone and occasionally joint fusion is required.

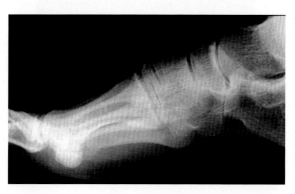

Fig. 9.2 Lateral radiograph with minimal osteophyte formation

Key points

- Tarsal bosses are a common cause of pain in the midfoot.
- Minor cases can be managed with attention to footwear.
- Large bumps may cause genuine problems and surgery with excision of the underlying bone may be necessary.
- Care is required during surgery to avoid the medial dorsal cutaneous nerve.

Further reading

Parker RG (2005) Dorsal foot pain due to compression of the deep peroneal nerve by exostosis of the metatarsocuneiform joint. Journal of the American Podiatric Association 95:455–8.

Case 10

A 50-year-old man presented with a swelling on the outside of his right foot. At times it reached 'the size of a golf ball' (Fig. 10.1). Normally, when it reached that size he stated that his foot would become uncomfortable and he would have difficulty with shoe fitting. He would then resort to piercing the swelling with a pin, expressing a gelatinous fluid like 'egg white'. He wondered whether he might find a more permanent cure.

1. What is the 'egg white' fluid that is expressed from the swelling and therefore what is the diagnosis?
2. What is the aetiopathology of this condition?
3. What should be done for this patient?

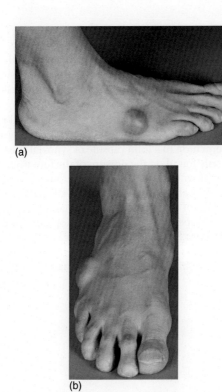

Fig. 10.1 (a, b) Swelling on the lateral aspect of the right foot

Ganglion

1. The description of the fluid is characteristic of synovial fluid, suggesting a ganglion cyst. A ganglion presents as a swelling that is soft, fluctuant and compressible. The size of the lesion can fluctuate.

2. Ganglia are cystic lesions containing gelatinous fluid resulting from myxoid degeneration of connective tissue. They arise through herniation of a joint capsule or synovial sheath. They are commonly found on the dorsum of the foot because of the number of synovial sheaths passing around the ankle (Fig. 10.2). They also occur as pea-like swellings in the flexor tendon sheaths of the toes. When illuminated, these fluid-filled tumours will disperse light in contrast to opaque solid masses. The ganglion cyst has variable appearance on ultrasound but MRI demonstrates a well-defined lesion with water-equivalent signal intensity (high on T2-weighted images).

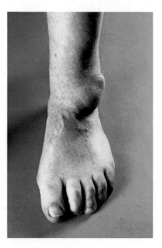

Fig. 10.2 Compressible swelling on the anterior ankle

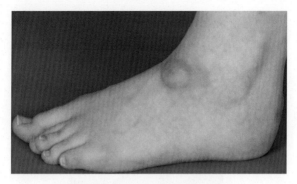

Fig. 10.3 Firm swelling on the anterior ankle

The lesion in Figure 10.3 looks similar to that shown above but in this case, the lesion was firm, adherent to the skin and non-compressible. This particular lesion did not illuminate and had low signal on T1- and T2-weighted MRI sequences. It was subsequently diagnosed as a benign fibroma but generally solid masses should be viewed with suspicion.

3. If asymptomatic and small, then ganglia are best left alone. Ganglia that become large or uncomfortable, as in the case illustrated above, should be aspirated to provide the patient with at least temporary relief of the symptoms. The patient should, however, be informed that the rate of recurrence from aspiration alone will be in excess of 70%. This may be reduced by corticosteroid injection although some skin discolouration and possible subcutaneous fat atrophy is to be expected. Excision of the lesion (Fig. 10.4) will provide a more certain result, provided that care is taken to ensure that the entire cyst wall is removed and any underlying bone protuberance from periosteal trauma or joint degeneration is excised.

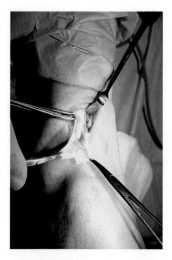

Fig. 10.4 Surgical excision of a dorsal ankle ganglion

Evidence

Low-level evidence from an observational study suggests that surgical intervention of ganglia results in less recurrence (11%) compared with conservative treatment consisting of aspiration and aspiration combined with steroid injection (63%).

Key points

- Ganglia are common on the dorsum of the foot.
- Ganglia are benign lesions, containing gelatinous fluid, arising through herniation of a joint capsule or tendon sheath.
- Asymptomatic lesions do not require intervention.
- Large and uncomfortable swellings can be aspirated, but excision will often be required.

Further reading

Foo LF, Raby N (2005) Tumours and tumour-like lesions of the foot and ankle. Clinical Radiology 60(3):308–32.

Kirby EJ, Shereff MJ, Lewis MM (1989) Soft-tissue tumors and tumor-like lesions of the foot. An analysis of eighty-three cases. Journal of Bone and Joint Surgery 71:459–65.

Pontious J, Good J, Maxian SH (1999) Ganglions of the foot and ankle: a retrospective analysis of 63 procedures. Journal of the American Podiatric Medical Association 89(4):163–8.

Case 11

This middle-aged woman has a long-standing lesion on the plantar surface of her great toe (Figs 11.1a and b). The lesion has slowly become bigger over several years but, despite its size, it has not been particularly troublesome. Recently, she traumatized the lesion and it was painful and so this encouraged her to seek treatment to have the lesion removed. The 2 × 1.2 × 1.2 cm lesion had a firm consistency and was painful to touch. It was excised with a clear margin of normal tissue. Figure 11.3 shows the microscopic appearance.

This lesion on the sole of the foot had a rather unusual appearance.

1. How would you describe this lesion to a colleague?
2. What might it be?
3. Discuss the histology shown in Figure 11.2.

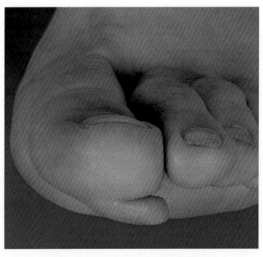

Fig. 11.1 (a) End-on view of great toe

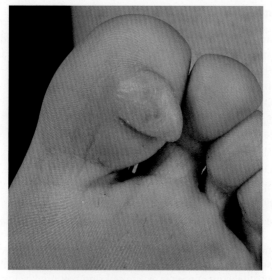

Fig. 11.1 (b) Plantar view of great toe

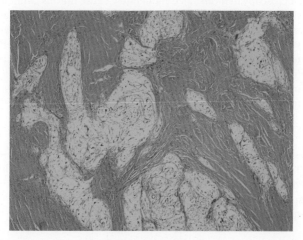

Fig. 11.2 Photomicrograph of lesion

Neurothekeoma (nerve sheath myxoma)

1. Examination reveals a flesh-coloured, well-circumscribed dome-shaped papule (see Fig. 11.1b). The lesion is well vascularized and Figure 11.1a shows that it is pedunculated.

2. Differential diagnoses include:
   - Dermal inclusion cyst
   - Epidermoid cyst
   - Neurilemomma
   - Neurofibroma
   - Dermatofibroma
   - Spitz naevus
   - Fibrokeratoma (garlic clove tumour)

   The actual diagnosis for this lesion was a neurothekeoma-myxoid variant (nerve sheath myxoma), a benign soft tissue tumour of the dermis originating from nerve sheath cells. It is a rare condition that is seldom seen in the lower limb. Neurothekeoma presents as a raised skin-coloured lesion, averaging 1 cm in diameter. The lesion is non-invasive and is not prone to metastasis.

3. Microscopy demonstrated moderately dense fibrous connective tissue containing circumscribed cell-poor nodules. These have a myxoid background and contain scattered spindle-shaped and stellate cells with relatively bland nuclear features. These cells react positively with antibodies to s-100 protein and epithelial membrane antigen (EMA) but not CD57 antigen, smooth muscle actin, desmin or CD10 antigen. These features are typical for a neurothekeoma, myxoid variant.

Key points

- A neurothekeoma is a benign soft tissue tumour of the dermis originating from nerve sheath cells.
- Excision of the lesion and histological confirmation are required.

Further reading

Papadopoulos EJ, Cohen PR, Hebert AA (2004) Neurothekeoma: report of a case in an infant and review of the literature. Journal of the American Academy of Dermatology 50(1):129–34.

Persich G, Portela M (2004) Neurothekeoma in the foot: a rare occurrence. Journal of the American Podiatric Medicine Association 94(1):59–60.

Case 12

For six months a 40-year-old events manager complained that she had experienced pain under the arch of her foot, particularly troublesome when wearing her ski boots. She reports that her father and brother have nodules on the palms of their hands. Inspection reveals a lesion, shown in Figure 12.1.

1. This lump is painful. What would be a reasonable differential diagnosis?
2. There are certain factors predisposing to lesions of this type; can you name them?
3. Assuming that the lump was excised, what might be the end result?

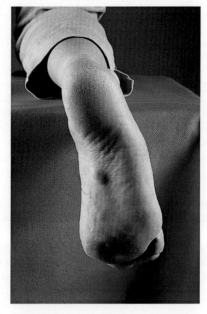

Fig. 12.1 Lesion in the sole of the left foot

Plantar fibroma

1. The lesion shown is typical of a nodule arising within the plantar fascia (Fig. 12.2). There are actually very few other conditions which might produce a similarly tender nodule. Granulomas may occur around a foreign body, but the patient is usually aware of preceding trauma. The only other lesion of note, assuming that there is no underlying bony abnormality, is a neurilemmoma (Schwannoma: tumour of a peripheral nerve sheath) as shown in Figure 12.3.

2. Plantar fibromatosis is analogous to palmar fibromatosis (Dupuytren's disease) and it is generally accepted that they are one and the same condition. Histological analysis in the early stages will identify arrays of myofibroblasts, producing a lesion that tends to be fairly soft and may be exquisitely tender. At this stage, care has to be taken to ensure that the lesion is not mistaken for a fibrosarcoma. With maturity, these characteristics change as the nodule becomes much firmer because of a decrease in cell density and a laying down of collagen.

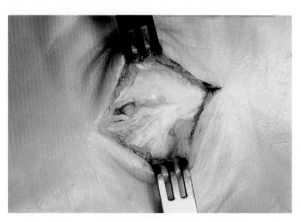

Fig. 12.2 Plantar fibroma

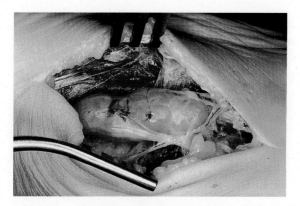

Fig. 12.3 Plantar neurilemmoma

The most common identifiable factor predisposing to a plantar lesion is probably trauma. This may simply have been a tearing of the fibres of the ligament, similar to that causing plantar fasciitis, or a direct laceration. The fact that direct trauma will not always cause fibroma formation indicates that the patient must also have a predisposition to the condition. A genetic link is fairly well established, certainly in patients with a Dupuytren's palmar contracture. Affected subjects will often have a familial tendency to the condition and there is also an association with idiopathic epilepsy and excessive alcohol intake.

3. A conservative approach to treatment is generally recommended. With the passage of time the lesions become less acutely tender, although they never alter much in size. Steroid infiltration may reduce perinodular inflammation, but will not shrink the lesion per se. If a lesion becomes large then surgical excision may be requested. The patient should be warned that recurrence is likely, especially if the nodules are multiple, bilateral or occur in patients with a strong family history. Since the lesion usually infiltrates the dermis a skin graft may be required.

Key points

- Plantar fibromatosis is common in Caucasians.
- The lesion consists of myofibroblasts linked to extracellular filaments.
- Treatment should be conservative if possible.
- Recurrence is frequent after surgical resection.

Further reading

De Palma L, Santucci A, Gigante A, Di Giulio A, Carloni S (1999) Plantar fibromatosis: an immunohistochemical and ultrastructural study. Foot and Ankle International 20:253–7.

Fetsch JF, Laskin WB, Miettinen M (2005) Palmar-plantar fibromatosis in children and pre-adolescents: a clinicopathologic study of 56 cases with newly recognized demographics and extended follow-up information. American Journal of Surgical Pathology 29(8):1095–105.

Sammarco GJ, Mangone PG (2000) Classification and treatment of plantar fibromatosis. Foot and Ankle International 21:563–9.

Case 13

A teenage girl presents with a painful big toenail. The pain is exacerbated with certain footwear and with direct pressure on the nail plate. The nail plate has separated from the nail bed and the lesion has been discharging (Fig. 13.1a, b). As a result, she has received two courses of antibiotics. This girl's mother is convinced that this is an ingrowing toenail and she has sought advice from a podiatrist.

1. Why is this girl's mother wrong in her assessment of this toenail problem and what are your differential diagnoses?
2. What is the cause of this toenail condition?
3. How would you confirm your diagnosis?
4. What is the correct management of this condition?

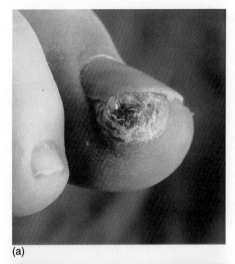

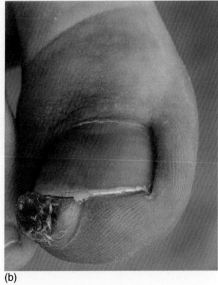

Fig. 13.1 (a, b) Raised nail plate

Subungual exostosis

1. A firm swelling appears under the nail plate, raising it from the nail bed. Compare this with the ingrowing toenail in Figure 28.1, where hypergranulation tissue forms at the nail folds. This therefore is a subungual exostosis. Other differential diagnoses would be a subungual wart, corn, malignant melanoma or periungual fibroma (Fig. 13.2).

2. Subungual exostosis is a benign tumour of trabecular bone with a fibrocartilage cap. It presents most frequently in teenagers and young adults. Exostoses are reputed to be caused by trauma, but there is no strong evidence for this and most patients do not report a traumatic incident. In 70% of cases the great toe is affected.

3. Diagnosis is confirmed by radiograph. Histology demonstrates a stalk of normal trabecular bone capped with fibrocartilage (Fig. 13.3).

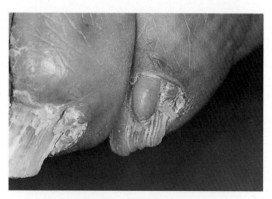

Fig. 13.2 Periungual fibroma of proximal nail fold

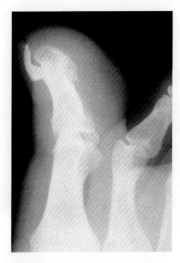

Fig. 13.3 Lateral radiograph of hallux

4. Complete surgical excision is the treatment of choice. This can be performed on a day case basis using a ring block anaesthetic (Fig. 13.4) and a tourniquet around the toe. The toenail is completely removed, preferably without disturbing the nail matrix. The stalk of the exostosis is removed with bone rongeurs or a small osteotome, so that bone is removed from below the level of the normal periosteum. Sufficient bone must be removed to avoid recurrence (reported to be as high as 15% within 1 year). The wound should be left open and allowed to close by secondary intention.

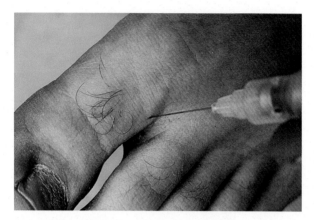

Fig. 13.4 Technique of local anaesthetic injection of the hallux

---

Clinical tip: technique of hallux injection

Use plain solutions of 1% or 2% lignocaine hydrochloride 2–4 ml (or 0.5% bupivacaine hydrochloride 1–2 ml). A dental needle (see Fig. 13.4) is ideal but failing this, a small-diameter (blue) needle should be used. Identify the MTP and the IP joints and find the midpoint of the proximal phalanx. Always inject the lateral side of the toe first (see Fig. 13.4), as this is less painful. Introduce the needle at an angle of 60° to the skin and insert the needle to the plantar side of the toe. Inject 0.5–1 ml of anaesthetic plantarward and the same dorsally. Repeat on the medial side.

Key points

- The great toenail is affected in 70% of cases.
- Pain arises where the nail plate becomes raised and distorted.
- Radiographs confirm the diagnosis.
- Surgical excision is the treatment of choice.

Further reading

David D, Cohen P (1996) Subungual exostosis: case report and review of the literature. Paediatric Dermatology 13:212–18.

De Berker D, Langtry J (1999) Treatment of subungual exostoses by elective day case surgery. British Journal of Dermatology 140:915–18.

Section 3

Orthopaedics

Case 14

A 45-year-old ex-ballerina presents with a painful great toe and dorsal swelling as shown in Figure 14.1.

1. This patient had virtually no movement at her MTP joint. What terms are used to describe restricted movement at the first MTP joint?

2. Young patients with this condition often report that they have participated in competitive sport. Which sports are particularly bad for your toe and what other conditions will lead to the radiographic appearances shown in Figure 14.2?

3. What functional variations may predispose a patient to this condition?

4. Outline an appropriate grading system.

5. What conservative treatments might lessen this patient's pain?

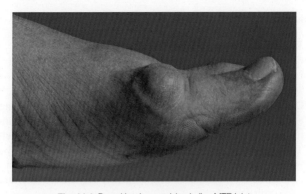

Fig. 14.1 Dorsal bunion overlying hallux MTP joint

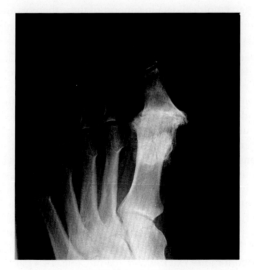

Fig. 14.2 Radiograph of great toe

1. The dorsal prominence seen is indicative of underlying degenerative osteoarthritis and dorsal osteophyte formation. Limitation and absence of movement are termed hallux 'limitus' and 'rigidus', respectively.

2. Degenerative joint arthritis arises from direct cartilage damage, and players of any sport who kick a ball repetitively are prone to hallux rigidus. In American footballers the condition is labelled 'turf toe'. Sepsis, inflammatory arthritis or excessive repetitive weight transfer (a similar factor to that causing osteochondritis of the second metatarsal head) all potentially lead to the same end result.

3. Metatarsus elevatus and first ray hypermobility, as occur secondary to abnormal stance phase pronation, are reportedly associated with an increased risk of acquiring hallux rigidus, although empirical data in support of these theories are lacking.

4. A number of grading systems are available for hallux rgidus. A five-point scoring system is provided in Table 14.1.

5. Two factors produce symptoms and it may be important to address one or both of these. Firstly, as osteoarthritis of the MTP joint progresses, the joint space narrows, which leads to tendon and ligament contractures and associated stiffness. Secondly, osteophytes form around the margins of the joint, particularly dorsally and laterally, leading to a mechanical block to extension and sometimes hallux flexus.

    Transient benefits may be gained from simple conservative treatments. Non-steroidal anti-inflammatory drugs, rest and elevation of the foot may all help if the toe is particularly sore. Intra-articular steroid injections provide short-term pain relief, but a rigid insole should restrict joint movement sufficiently to lessen pain (Fig. 14.3). A rocker on the sole is also worth fitting as this acts to offload the first metatarsal head by reducing the need for joint extension at 'toe-off' (Fig. 14.4). If these treatments fail, then patients will generally consider surgery.

Table 14.1 A five-point grading system for hallux rigidus (after Coughlin & Shurnas 2003)

Grade	Dorsiflexion	Radiographic findings	Clinical findings
0	40–60° and/or 10–20% loss compared with normal side	Normal	No pain: only stiffness and loss of motion on examination
1	30–40° and/or 20–50% loss compared with normal side	Dorsal osteophyte is main finding, minimal joint space narrowing, minimal periarticular sclerosis, minimal flattening of metatarsal head	Mild or occasional pain and stiffness, pain at extremes of dorsiflexion and/or plantarflexion on examination
2	10–30° and/or 50–75% loss compared with normal side	Dorsal, lateral and possibly medial osteophytes giving flattened appearance to metatarsal head, no more than ¼ of dorsal joint involved on lateral radiograph, mild to moderate joint space narrowing and sclerosis, sesamoids not usually involved	Moderate to severe pain and stiffness that may be constant: pain occurs just before maximum dorsiflexion and maximum plantarflexion on examination
3	≤10° and/or 75–100% loss compared with normal side. There is notable loss of MTP plantarflexion as well (often ≤10° of plantarflexion)	Same as in grade 2 but with substantial narrowing, possibly periarticular cystic changes, more than ¼ of dorsal joint space involved on lateral radiograph, sesamoids enlarged and/or cystic and/or irregular	Nearly constant pain and substantial stiffness at extremes of range of motion but not at mid-range
4	Same as in grade 3	Same as in grade 3	Same criteria as grade 3 but there is definite pain at mid-range of passive motion

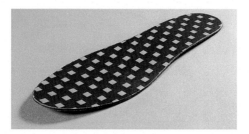

Fig. 14.3 Carbonflex insole

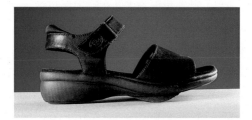

Fig. 14.4 Rocker sole

Evidence

Patients with mild (grade I) hallux rigidus gained symptomatic relief for a median of 6 months following injection of steroid and manipulation of the joint.

Key points

- Hallux limitus/rigidus is a degenerative condition.
- Painful joint extension prevents normal gait.
- A scoring system is available to aid decision making.
- In-shoe orthoses should be considered in grade I or grade II hallux limitus/rigidus.
- A rocker sole may be helpful.

Further reading

Coughlin MJ, Shurnas PS (2003) Hallux rigidus. Grading and long term results of operative treatment. Journal of Bone and Joint Surgery 85-A(11):2072–88.

Horton GA, Park Y-W, Myerson MS (1999) Role of metatarsus primus elevatus in the pathogenesis of hallux rigidus. Foot and Ankle International 20:777–80.

Smith RW, Katchis SD, Ayson LC (2000) Outcomes in hallux rigidus patients treated nonoperatively: a long-term follow-up study. Foot and Ankle International 21:906–13.

Solan MC, Calder JD, Bendall SP (2001) Manipulation and injection for hallux rigidus. Is it worthwhile? Journal of Bone and Joint Surgery 83-B(5):706–8.

Case 15

A distinctive bony prominence has developed overlying this lady's second metatarsal head (Fig. 15.1). She is 61 years old, retired and has a long-standing history of pain in her right foot. On examination, movement at her MTP joint was severely restricted.

1. Given the objective symptoms, explain the presence of this dorsal prominence.
2. Does this condition only occur in adolescents?
3. Describe the pathology of the condition.
4. Do conservative measures have anything to offer this patient?
5. What are the surgical options?

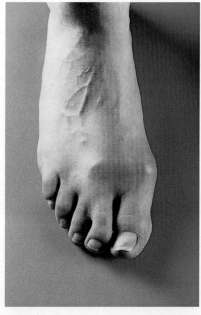

Fig. 15.1 Clinical appearance of the foot showing distinctive dorsal prominence

Freiberg's infraction

1. Osteochondritis of the second metatarsal head, termed Freiberg's infraction, is a common, crushing-type osteochondritis leading to avascular necrosis. It most commonly arises in adolescent girls but may also affect boys. Although this patient does remember an episode of a painful foot as a youngster, she did not present until later life when she developed pain in her second MTP joint.

2. No. Most of the literature describes the cause as an insult to the blood supply of the open epiphysis of the metatarsal head. However, Figures 15.2a and 15.2b show radiographs of a 64-year-old man taken 4 years ago for a coincidental injury and then this year for recent forefoot pain. Clearly this shows the development of a 'new Freiberg's' and is evidence that avascular necrosis of the metatarsal head can occur in later life.

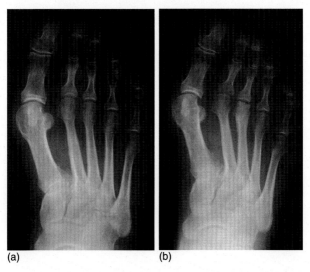

(a)   (b)

Fig. 15.2 (a, b) Radiograph of 64-year-old man: normal third MTP joint

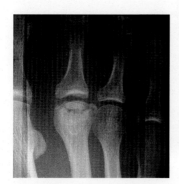

Fig. 15.3 AP radiograph: infraction of second metatarsal head

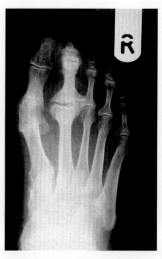

Fig. 15.4 AP radiograph showing replacement arthoplasty of second MTP joint

3. The head of the metatarsal progressively collapses or 'infracts' into the avascular segment (Fig. 15.3). This leads to flattening of the metatarsal articular surface, head compression and loss of joint space. The later changes are those of secondary osteoarthritis (Fig. 15.4). The classic description of the pathology of Freiberg's was provided by Smillie In 1967 and the five stages are summarized in Table 15.1.

4. A rocker sole (Fig. 14.4) may be advantageous as it will aid dorsiflexion of the foot. Local injections of corticosteroid provide only short-term symptomatic relief.

5. In the older patient, where degenerative changes are the cause of discomfort, either a proximal hemiphalangectomy or, as in this case, a joint replacement arthroplasty will be required (Fig. 15.5). In younger patients, Gauthier's procedure restores joint congruity by rotating the 'normal' dorsal cartilage onto the articulating surface (Fig. 15.6).

Table 15.1 Staging of Freiberg's infraction (after Smillie 1967):

Stage 1	A fissure fracture develops in the ischaemic epiphysis
Stage II	Absorption of bone has taken place and the central portion begins to sink into the head, altering the contour of the articular cartilage
Stage III	Further absorption has occurred and the central portion sinks into the head leaving projections on either side. The plantar articular cartilage remains intact.
Stage IV	The plantar isthmus of articular cartilage has given way and the loose body separated. Fractures of the lateral and dorsal projections have occurred. Restoration of the anatomy is no longer possible. The epiphysis is probably closed at this stage.
Stage V	Final stage of flattening, deformity and arthrosis.

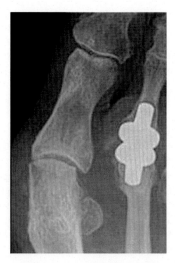

Fig. 15.5 Replacement arthroplasty

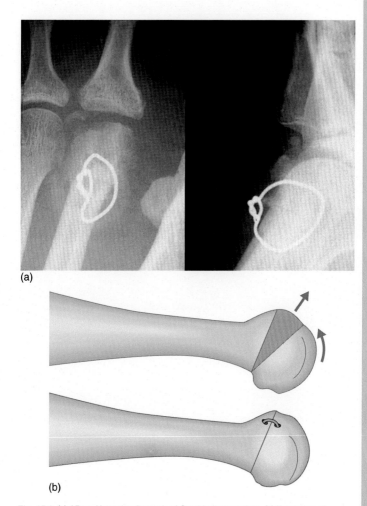

(a)

(b)

Fig. 15.6 (a) AP and lateral radiograph of Gauthier's procedure. (b) Illustration of Gauthier's procedure (lateral view).

Key points

- Freiberg's infraction occurs mainly in adolescence but not exclusively.
- The condition is an avascular necrosis of the metatarsal head.
- Secondary osteoarthritis always develops.
- In older patients, replacement or resection arthroplasty may be necessary.

Further reading

Hay SM, Smith TWD (1992) Freiberg's disease: an unusual presentation at the age of 50 years. The Foot 2:176–8.

Smillie IS (1967) Treatment of Freiberg's infraction. Proceedings of the Royal Society of Medicine 60:29–31.

Smith TWD, Stanley D, Rowley DI (1991) Treatment of Freiberg's disease: a new operative technique. Journal of Bone and Joint Surgery 73-B:129–30.

Townshend DN, Greiss M (2007) Total ceramic arthroplasty for painful, destructive disorders of the lesser metatarso-phalangeal joints. The Foot 17(2):73–5.

Case 16

A middle-aged lady complains of a painful second toe when walking. Her shoe has rubbed on the toe for some years.

1. Which digital deformity is this (Fig. 16.1) and what causes it?
2. What treatment options will relieve the pressure over the dorsum of the toe?
3. What clinical test indicates instability at the MTP joint? How is joint subluxation addressed?
4. Is there any specific therapy that might prevent the deformity recurring following surgery?

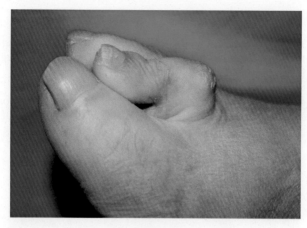

Fig. 16.1 Second toe deformity

Hammer toe

1. The photograph shows the typical appearance of hammering of the second toe. It is potentially serious, particularly if healing is compromised as shown in Figure 16.2. This condition is distinguishable from claw toe (Fig. 16.3) in which there is greater flexion of the distal interphalangeal (IP) joint and dorsal subluxation of the MTP joint. In mallet toe the distal IP joint only is flexed (Fig. 16.4).

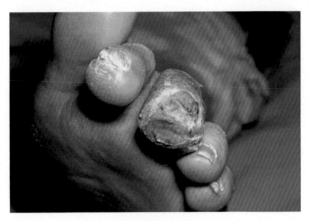

Fig. 16.2 Terminal ulceration

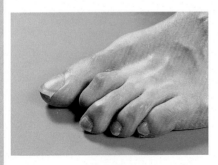

Fig. 16.3 Claw toe

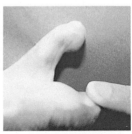

Fig. 16.4 Mallet toe

Hammer toe is often familial and usually gradually progressive from a young age. Frequently the second toe and/or the second metatarsal is abnormally long, i.e. the foot is 'index minus' or of 'Greek' type, respectively, and such a deformity leads to increased tension, at least on the medial aspect of the plantar aponeurosis. Direct pull onto the plantar plate and flexor tendon sheath at the level of the MTP joint explains the joint flexion. In the elderly, since the aponeurosis stretches out with age, there does have to be some dorsiflexion of the proximal phalanx before flexion of the PIP joint will occur.

2. PIP joint fusion is probably the most commonly performed surgical procedure for hammer toe. Articular cartilage is removed from the head of the proximal phalanx and from the base of the middle phalanx and the surfaces apposed. The fusion is held with a fine Kirschner wire or a biodegradable pin. Hohman has recommended excision of the head of the proximal phalanx and reefing of the dorsal extensor tendon only. We have generally found that this produces an inferior result to fusion, as some patients will experience continuing discomfort from the mobile joint. Hemiphalangectomy (Fig. 16.5) may leave a redundant and shortened digit and amputation produces gapping which in the case of the second toe will cause the hallux to move across into valgus (Fig. 16.6).

3. Pain elicited at the MTP joint on 'drawing' the toe dorsally on the metatarsal will signify joint instability. Resection of the IP joint does produce a relative lengthening of the dorsal extensor tendon that may be sufficient to prevent subluxation of the proximal phalanx dorsally on the metatarsal. If not, it is worthwhile performing a dorsal capsulotomy of the MTP joint and possibly also a transfer of the dorsal extensor tendon to the flexor below the metatarsal head. If this is still inadequate then a Weil's sliding osteotomy may be required (Figs 16.7, 16.8).

4. After PIP joint arthrodesis it is worthwhile prescribing a metatarsal dome insole to support the second metatarsal head (Fig. 16.9).

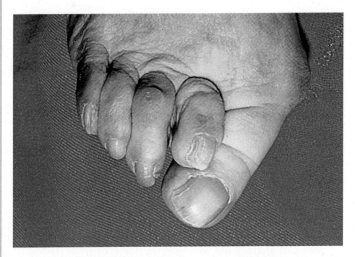

Fig. 16.5 Appearance after proximal hemiphalangectomy

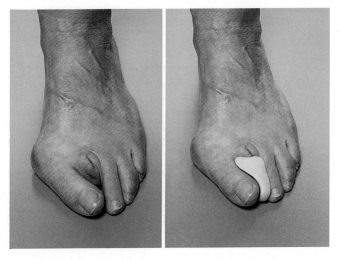

Fig. 16.6 Hallux valgus deformity after second toe amputation with and without spacer

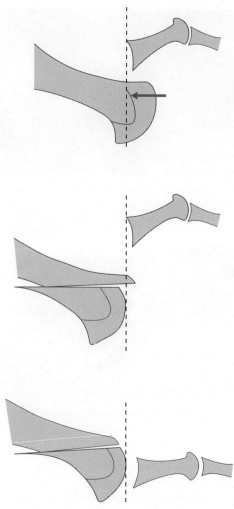

Fig. 16.7 Weil's osteotomy

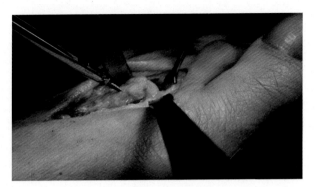

Fig. 16.8 Weil's osteotomy held with a 'snap-off' screw

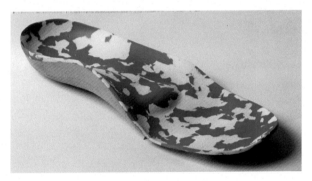

Fig. 16.9 Metatarsal dome support

Key points

- Dorsal and terminal corns will arise secondary to fixed flexion of the PIP toe joint.
- Operative treatment is generally beneficial.
- PIP joint fusion is probably the most common procedure performed.
- A metatarsal dome support may be helpful.

Further reading

American College of Foot and Ankle Surgeons (1999) Hammer toe syndrome. Journal of Foot and Ankle Surgery 38:166–78.

Harmonson JK, Harkless LB (1996) Operative procedures for the correction of hammer toe, claw toe, and mallet toe: a literature review. Clinics in Podiatric Medicine and Surgery 13:211–20.

Trnka H-J, Gebhard C, Muhlbauer M, Ivanic G, Ritschl P (2002) The Weil osteotomy for treatment of dislocated lesser metatarsophalangeal joints: good outcome in 21 patients with 42 osteotomies. Acta Orthopaedica Scandinavica 73:190–4.

Case 17

A 76-year-old ex-army major presented with a request for new shoes. He stated that his feet had always been broad and that they had not inhibited his military service (Fig. 17.1).

Earlier in the same clinic a 45-year-old patient had presented with a similarly broad foot (Fig. 17.2).

1. What is the aetiology of polydactyly and is there a common pattern?
2. How will treatment vary for the different types of anomaly?
3. Would there be any indication for surgery in this elderly man?
4. What term is used to describe the enlarged toe shown and what treatment options might be considered?

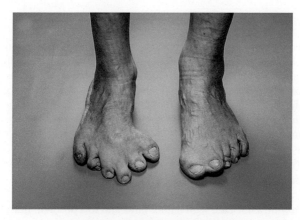

Fig. 17.1 Congenital forefoot deformity

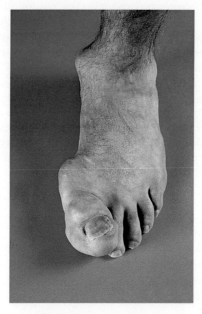

Fig. 17.2 Great toe hypertrophy

Polydactyly and macrodactyly

1. Polydactyly occurs either as an autosomal dominant mutation of a single gene, or a part of a syndrome of congenital anomalies arising from multiple gene mutations. Most frequently as a result of duplication of the fifth toe (up to 80%) or, as in this case, of the first ray. Middle toe duplication is much less common. The duplication may involve any part of the involved digit or the metatarsal. In this case the phalanges were duplex (Fig. 17.3).
2. Treatment of polydactyly is generally straightforward. The smallest digit, which may well be rudimentary, should be excised and the skin carefully closed by direct suture or rotational flaps as necessary. Preaxial (hallux) duplication may be associated with hallux varus and this problem must be addressed separately.
3. This elderly gentleman had never suffered any impairment of foot function as a result of his broad forefeet. Indeed, he had served in the army throughout the war, passing all the fitness tests. There would be absolutely no indication now to offer any form of treatment other than custom-made footwear.
4. Metatarsal or phalangeal duplication may lead to gigantism, but more commonly an entire ray is enlarged. (Fig. 17.4).

The soft tissue swelling observed was typical of that occuring in both classic gigantism, from neurofibromatosis, and in patients with a locally hyper dynamic circulation secondary to arteriovenous malformations. In fact, in this case there was evidence of excess fat deposition within the marrow and the patient was diagnosed as suffering from macrodystrophia lipomatosa. The disproportionate increase in fibroadipose tissue is a form of hamartoma.

Key points

- Postaxial polydactyly is most common.
- Indications for surgery may be functional or cosmetic.
- The least functional digit should be excised.
- Digital gigantism may occur in association with neurofibromatosis.

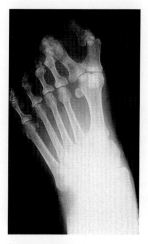

Fig. 17.3 Polydactyly: AP radiograph of left foot

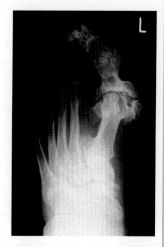

Fig. 17.4 Gigantism: AP radiograph showing widening of the first ray

Further reading

Chang CH, Kumar SJ, Riddle EC, Glutting J (2002) Macrodactyly of the foot. Journal of Bone and Joint Surgery 84-A:1189–94.

Phelps DA, Grogan DP (1985) Polydactyly of the foot. Journal of Pediatric Orthopedics 5:446–51.

Case 18

A 66-year-old woman presents with a tender bunion. Examination reveals a large bursal swelling and some hammering of the lesser digits (Figs 18.1, 18.2). She stated that the bunion had progressively enlarged over a few years.

1. What is the probable underlying cause of this lady's hallux valgus?
2. What factors have led to the hammering of this lady's lesser toes? If the second digit had been overriding, might amputation have been worthwhile?
3. In this case the patient had just recovered from a heart attack and did not wish to consider any form of surgery. What conservative measures might help to relieve her discomfort?

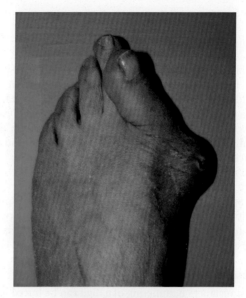

Fig. 18.1 Enlarged hallux bursa

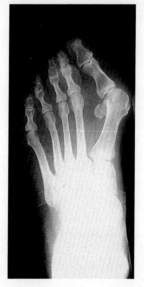

Fig. 18.2 Standing AP radiograph

Aetiology of hallux valgus

1. Many factors have been considered to be causative of hallux valgus. Probably the least important of these is the 'wearing of tight-fitting shoes'. Foot pronation, together with metatarsus primus varus, is generally evident in most patients presenting with 'bunions'. Lesser factors almost certainly include an abnormally acute cuneiform/first metatarsal angle and an insufficiency of the intermetatarsal band between the first and second metatarsal heads.

   Once the hallux has deviated laterally, the medial capsule of the MTP joint will be stretched and the sesamoids pulled laterally away from their normal plantar articulation on the underside of the first metatarsal head. The hallux deviation will be accentuated by the pull of the long flexor and extensor tendons, and the joint reaction forces created serve to push the metatarsal head even further medially.

2. In most instances hammering of a digit can be traced to a relative discrepancy in the length of the adjacent digits. It is particularly relevant if the patient has a 'Greek' type foot with an excessively long second metatarsal.

   Amputation is contraindicated even if the second toe is overriding the hallux. Removal of the second toe serves only to accentuate any hallux valgus and allows the sesamoids to displace even further laterally. The patient would then tend to offload the first ray by taking more weight on the lateral side of her foot.

3. Many elderly patients have lived with their foot deformities for many years. It is essential to provide comfortable shoes and these must usually be made to measure. A toe box with sufficient depth to accommodate the overriding digits is required and a silastic toe spacer may help (Fig. 18.3).

Evidence

Three randomized trials have considered conservative treatment for hallux valgus. The evidence from these suggests that orthoses and night splints did not prevent a deterioration in hallux valgus angle, or lead to an improvement in functional outcome scores.

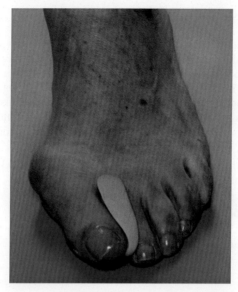

Fig. 18.3 Silastic toe spacer

Key points

- Surgery for hallux valgus is rarely obligatory.
- Wide-fitting shoes with sufficient room to accommodate the toes may be all that is required.
- Digit realignment generally requires metatarsal osteotomy.

Further reading

Bryant A, Tinley P, Singer K (2000) A comparison of radiographic measurements in normal, hallux valgus, and hallux limitus feet. Journal of Foot and Ankle Surgery 39:39–43.

Ferrari J, Higgins JPT, Prior TD (2007) Interventions for treating hallux valgus (abductovalgus) and bunions. Cochrane Database of Systematic Reviews, Issue 4. www.cochrane.org

Case 19

Runners can be plagued with a number of foot problems and the condition described here is particularly annoying. Left heel pain has troubled this 32-year-old long distance runner for some months. He reports no specific injury and describes his pain as sharp and usually worse first thing in the morning. With exercise, his pain diminishes, then recurs after rest. Examination reveals tenderness in the centre of his heel pad (Fig. 19.1) and a lateral radiograph is taken (Fig. 19.2).

1. Given the presenting symptoms, what is the most likely cause of this athlete's pain?
2. Why is pain worse first thing in the morning?
3. Describe the examination taking place in Figure 19.1.
4. What is shown in the radiograph in Figure 19.2 and what is its significance?
5. Outline a treatment plan for this patient.

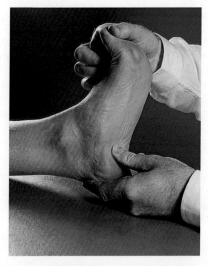

Fig. 19.1 Examination of the painful heel

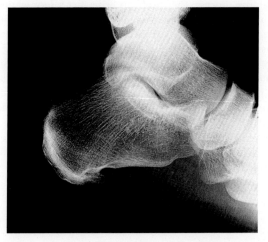

Fig. 19.2 Lateral radiograph of the left heel

Plantar fasciitis

1. Plantar fasciitis (also known as plantar heel pain syndrome or heel spur syndrome) is a common condition occurring at any time of life. It is seen in runners but also in less active patients. The 40-60 year age group is most frequently affected and the condition is more prevalent in obese individuals.

2. Pain after sleep and rest may be explained by contraction of the plantar fascia while the ankle is flexed, which is then suddenly stretched on weightbearing.

3. The exact site of tenderness is located by first applying tension to the plantar fascia. This is best done by dorsiflexion of the great toe (Hicks' windlass effect) and then running the thumb from distal to proximal along the medial aspect of its central portion (see Fig. 19.1). Firm pressure is then applied with a thumb over the medial calcaneal tuberosity and the pain elicited is diagnostic of the condition.

4. The significance of a plantar spur, as shown in Figure 19.2, is not clear. They are common in the general population, increasing in frequency with age (they occur in up to 16% of those over 50 years). Heel spurs are likely to be part of a reparative process. They probably arise after minor tearing of the plantar fascia's attachment onto the heel which causes bleeding and heterotopic ossification. In general, heel spurs are considered a normal variant and an insignificant finding when they are small, well defined and with smooth, regular cortical contours. X-rays to confirm a diagnosis of plantar fasciitis are not routinely indicated. Ultrasound scans are more useful, demonstrating increased thickness (> 5 mm) and oedema of the plantar fascia.

5. Plantar heel pain syndrome is self-limiting; 80% of cases resolve within 12 months but a number of therapies are advocated during the painful stages.

Evidence

A systematic review of 19 RCTs for the Cochrane Library concluded that there was limited evidence upon which to base clinical practice. This systematic review did establish that steroid injections are useful in the short term but only to a small degree. There was limited evidence that stretching exercises and heel pads are associated with better outcomes than custom-made orthoses in people who stand for more than 8 hours per day. There are no RCTs evaluating surgery or radiotherapy.

In recent years, extracorporeal shock wave therapy (ESWT) has emerged as a popular alternative to surgery for patients with chronic plantar fasciitis (Fig. 19.3). Some RCTs comparing shock wave therapy to placebo therapy support this mode of treatment, but a meta-analysis of 11 of these trials is equivocal.

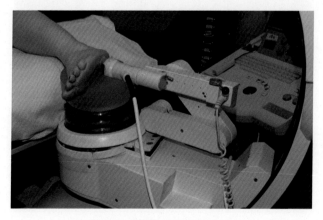

Fig. 19.3 ESWT applied to the heel

Clinical tip

We locate the site of maximal tenderness, then insert the needle at an angle to the skin until bone is met. The needle is then withdrawn slightly, the syringe aspirated and the solution injected: methyl prednisolone 0.5 ml (40 mg) and lignocaine hydrochloride 1 ml 2% (Fig. 19.4).

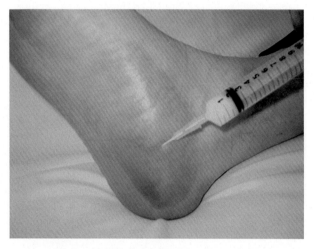

Fig. 19.4 Injection of corticosteroid for plantar fasciitis

Key points

- Plantar heel pain syndrome is typically seen as an overuse injury in runners or in well-built patients of middle age.
- Calcaneal spurs are common and are the result, rather than the cause, of plantar heel pain syndrome.
- Injections of corticosteroid appear to help, at least in the short term.
- A variety of orthoses may be helpful during the painful phase of this self-limiting condition.

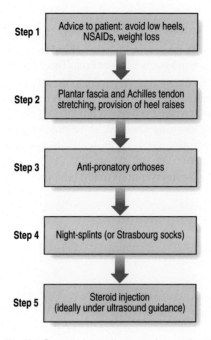

Step 1	Advice to patient: avoid low heels, NSAIDs, weight loss
Step 2	Plantar fascia and Achilles tendon stretching, provision of heel raises
Step 3	Anti-pronatory orthoses
Step 4	Night-splints (or Strasbourg socks)
Step 5	Steroid injection (ideally under ultrasound guidance)

Fig. 19.5 Suggested stepwise approach to treatment

Further reading

Buchbinder R (2004) Plantar fasciitis. New England Journal of Medicine 351:834.

Buchbinder R, Ptasznik R, Gordon J, Buchanan J, Prabaharan V, Forbes A (2002) Ultrasound guided extracorporeal shockwave therapy for plantar fasciitis: a randomized controlled trial. Journal of the American Medical Association 288:1364–72.

Crawford F, Thomson C (2003) Interventions for treating plantar heel pain. Cochrane Database of Systematic Reviews, Issue 2.

Gibbon W, Long G (1999) Ultrasound of the plantar aponeurosis (fascia). Skeletal Radiology 28: 21–6.

Thomson CE, Crawford F, Murray G (2005) The effectiveness of extra corporeal shock wave therapy for plantar heel pain: a systematic review and meta-analysis. BMC Musculoskeletal Disorders 6: 19.

Case 20

A 45-year-old lady presents with pain behind her heel after country dancing. Inspection reveals heel swelling (Fig. 20.1).

1. What are the differential diagnoses of these swellings and what predisposing factors are relevant? Which common synonyms are used to describe swellings at this site?
2. Will simply inserting a heel lift in the shoe help?
3. Does this condition only occur in middle-aged women or can it affect children?
4. What operative interventions might be appropriate?

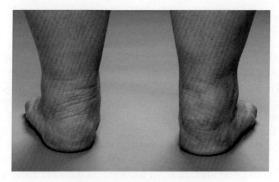

Fig. 20.1 Swelling posterior heels

Haglund's syndrome

1. Originally Haglund described a painful heel due to a combination of a bony prominence and low-backed shoes. Nowadays, 'Haglund's' encompasses retrocalcaneal bursa (bursa between calcaneus and Achilles tendon) and supracalcaneal bursa (subcutaneous bursa). Insertional Achilles tendinopathy develops with repetitive mechanical trauma and may be difficult to distinguish from retrocalcaneal bursa. All three conditions are associated with a prominent posterior superior border of the calcaneus aggravated by mechanically induced inflammation from footwear. In this case, there is pain and inflammation overlying a bony prominence at the posterolateral heel and a superficial bursitis has developed (Figs 20.2 to 20.3). This latter condition is also often referred to as a 'pump bump'. Occasionally inflammation at the posterior heel can be caused by inflammatory arthropathy.

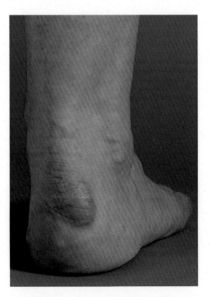

Fig. 20.2 Superficial Achilles bursitis

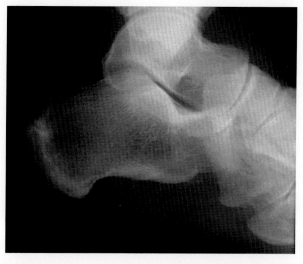

Fig. 20.3 Lateral heel radiograph showing large posterior calcaneal prominence and loose insertional spurs

2. Heel elevation would be appropriate for insertional Achilles tendinopathy. In this case the bursitis is aggravated by the patient's footwear. Therefore she requires advice regarding the type of shoes that she wears. Heel cups and soft pads applied to the heel or shoe will help with her discomfort.

3. Children are not commonly troubled with this condition. Sever's disease is a traction apophysitis at the posterior heel and it is treated with heel lifts and rest.

4. Steroid injections are not advocated for superficial bursitis. If symptoms persist despite conservative measures, then the prominence must be resected or a wedge osteotomy constructed to turn it in towards the talus (Fig. 20.4).

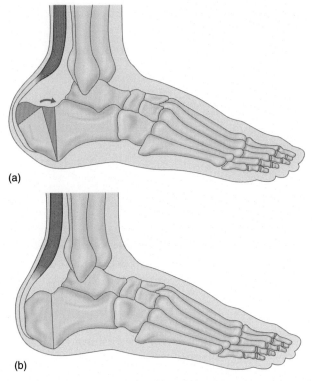

(a)

(b)

Fig. 20.4 (a, b) Dorsal calcaneal osteotomy

Key points

- Haglund's syndrome may include insertional Achilles tendinopathy, retrocalcaneal bursitis and superficial bursitis – 'pump bump'.
- Aspiration and steroid injection may be useful in retrocalcaneal bursitis but are never performed for superficial bursitis. Patients *must* be made aware of the potential risk of subsequent tendon rupture.
- Resection of a heel bump is generally possible through a direct lateral approach.

Further reading

Aldridge T (2004) Diagnosing heel pain in adults. American Family Physician 70(2):332–8.

Leitze Z, Sella EJ, Aversa JM (2003) Endoscopic decompression of the retrocalcaneal space. Journal of Bone and Joint Surgery 85-A:1488–96.

Mazzone M, McCue T (2002) Common conditions of the Achilles tendon. American Family Physician 65(9):1805–10.

Case 21

The patient in Case 14 continues to complain of severe pain despite use of a hallux limitus plate. It is suggested that osteophyte trimming might be helpful (Fig. 21.1).

1. What is this operation called?
2. Are there any other alternative simple surgical procedures?
3. What is the optimal angle of joint arthrodesis? Are there any contraindications to fusion?
4. Is there a place for joint arthroplasty?

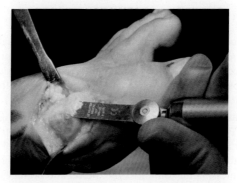

Fig. 21.1 Excision of dorsal osteophytes of the MTP joint

Surgery of hallux rigidus

1. Resection of the dorsal osteophytic lip is termed dorsal cheilectomy. Theoretically, the procedure allows the proximal phalanx to ride up over the metatarsal head in extension. In our experience patients only gain short-term benefit from this operation.

2. When arthritis is quite minor with minimal narrowing of the MTP joint space (grade 1 on a scale of 3) osteotomies of Weil or modified chevron type may be adequate (Table 21.1). These allow proximal displacement of the metatarsal head decompressing the joint. In 1958, Kessel and Bonney reported the use of a dorsiflexion osteotomy at the base of the proximal phalanx to relieve the pain of hallux rigidus in adolescents. Their patients retained plantarflexion of their toes but had lost dorsiflexion, probably because of a developmental elevation of their first metatarsal. Surgery transfers the arc of movement dorsally, improving toe function (Fig. 21.2). The condition is not common in adolescents and the operation is rarely performed.

3. Arthrodesis remains the most popular surgical procedure for hallux rigidus. Ideally the toe should be fused with 10-15° dorsiflexion relative to the sole of the foot, equating to a bone MTP angle of 20-25°. A flexion angle at the top end of this range is required in women wishing to wear a high-heeled shoe. The relief of their pain undoubtedly pleases many patients, but consequently there is complete loss of joint mobility and a long-term tendency for patients to overload the lateral side of

Table 21.1 Treatment options according to radiological grade

Grade 0	Grade 1	Grade 2	Grade 3
No osteophytes	Minimal joint space narrowing; dorsal osteophyte	Flattened metatarsal head; no sesamoid involvement	Substantial joint space narrowing; sesamoids arthritic
Release of plantar plate	Weil's osteotomy; modified chevron osteotomy	Dorsal cheilectomy	MTP fusion; MTP arthroplasty

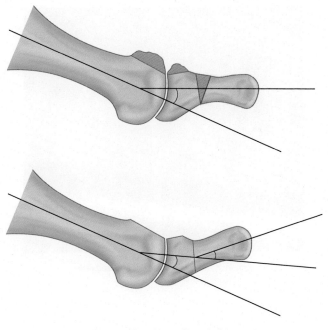

Fig. 21.2 Dorsal extension osteotomy

their feet. Arthritis of the IP joint is a contraindication to MTP fusion, as pain from the distal joint will become intolerable. Fusion of both joints is inadvisable as the patient will be left with neither proprioception nor toe-grip.

Several methods are commonly used to stabilize the arthrodesis until its union, but we have found that all of these will fail in some subjects, especially those with poor peripheral circulation. Indeed, the incidence of secondary surgery may be as high as 10% and patients should be forewarned. Plating (Fig. 21.3) and fusion by circlage wire and a crossed Kirschner wire (Fig. 21.4) are both effective and provide more rotational stability than insertion of a single cortical screw.

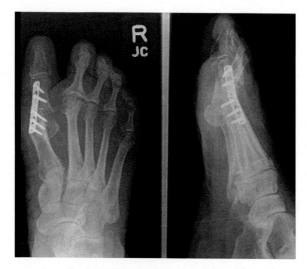

Fig. 21.3 MTP fusion using a contoured plate

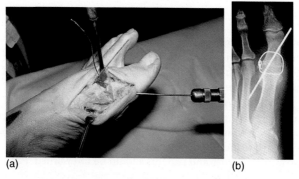

(a)   (b)

Fig. 21.4 (a, b) Joint arthrodesis using circlage wire

4. The most common alternative to fusion of the first MTP joint remains a resection arthroplasty (Keller's procedure). Postoperative function will be acceptable in the elderly, but many younger patients find that their shortened toe is floppy and that they greatly miss the inherent stability afforded by a normal hallux.

In the past few years, there has been a trend towards joint replacement rather than fusion. There have been reports of fairly good long-term results using both hinged and phalangeal peg silastic implants. Unfortunately, some patients develop severe granulomatous reactions to any silastic debris, causing device loosening and ultimately failure (Fig. 21.5). Total joint arthroplasty is a more attractive proposition. Reasonable functional results are now being reported from various implants on the market (Fig. 21.6). As with fusion, we have found that it may be at least 9 months after surgery before patients regain a normal gait.

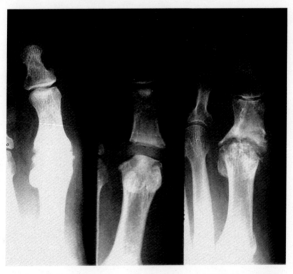

Fig. 21.5 Silastic hinge prosthesis at implantation and 15 years later

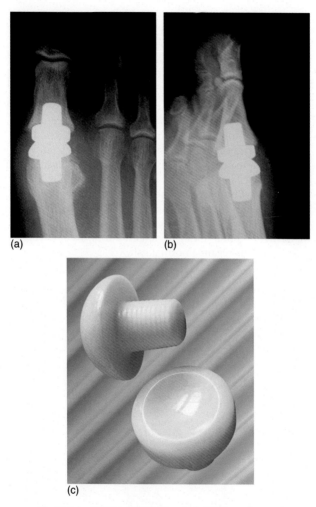

Fig. 21.6 (a-c) Mojé total joint arthroplasty (Ceramax, Germany)

Key points

- Fusion is the gold standard for treatment.
- IP arthritis is an absolute contraindication to MTP fusion.
- Total joint arthroplasty may be a valid alternative.

Evidence

One RCT compared MTP joint arthroplasty with fusion. At two year follow-up patients in both groups had benefited from surgery, but those who had a fusion had significantly less pain. The cost ratio was 2:1 in favour of arthrodesis.

Further reading

Gibson JNA, Thomson CE (2005) Arthrodesis or total replacement arthroplasty for hallux rigidus: a randomized controlled trial. Foot and Ankle 26:680–90.

Kessel L, Bonney G (1958) Hallux rigidus in the adolescent. Journal of Bone and Joint Surgery 40-B:668–73.

O'Doherty DP, Lowrie IG, Magnussen PA et al (1990) The management of the painful first metatarsophalangeal joint in the older patient: arthrodesis or Keller's arthroplasty? Journal of Bone and Joint Surgery 72-B:839–42.

Phillips JE, Hooper G (1986) A simple technique for arthrodesis of the first metatarsophalangeal joint. Journal of Bone and Joint Surgery 68-B:774–5.

Swanson AB (1972) Implant arthroplasty in disabilities of the great toe. In: Cacausland WR (ed) American Academy of Orthopaedic Surgeons Instructional Course Lectures XXI. St Louis, MO: CV Mosby, 227–35.

Case 22

Patients complaining of forefoot pain are often found to have callosities under their metatarsal heads. A 70-year-old man presents complaining that he feels he is 'walking on pebbles' (Fig. 22.1).

1. What factors might have contributed to the development of this condition?
2. Why did the callosities develop and what is the actual source of pain?
3. How might the surgeon endeavour to relieve the patient's symptoms if all conservative treatments have failed?
4. What long-term result may be expected from surgery?

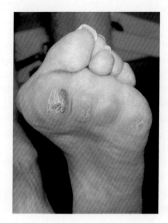

Fig. 22.1 Forefoot callosities

Metatarsalgia

1. This patient initially presented to his general practitioner
   with hammering of his toes. The significance of MTP joint
   subluxation (Fig. 22.2) was not recognized and an insole was
   of no benefit and not worn. It was only a matter of time before
   pressure callosities developed. Indeed, it might be argued that
   the hammering of the digits only arose because of alteration of
   the normal weight distribution across the forefoot as ageing
   occurred and the metatarsal heads splayed. Similar progressive
   deformity would have developed had the patient suffered from
   rheumatoid arthritis.

2. Callosities develop as the subcutaneous tissues underlying the
   metatarsal heads atrophy. These changes are exacerbated by
   displacement of the plantar fat pad distally. Pain arises from
   the effects of direct pressure on the sole, metatarsal bursitis and
   joint synovitis.

3. The fundamental objective of any surgery is to produce a
   smooth 'arc' across the metatarsal bed. This may be achieved by
   selective shortening of the lesser metatarsals, allowing

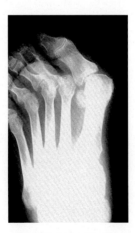

Fig. 22.2 Joint subluxation

the metatarsal heads to slide proximally. Clinical results from a Weil's osteotomy (see Fig. 16.7) are better than those from dorsal displacement of the metatarsal head as described by Helal. Usually, however, it is necessary to manufacture some form of procedure that will bring the plantar fat pad back into its rightful position. In this instance, the metatarsal condyles and proximal phalanges were resected through a dorsal approach (Fig. 22.3). It was felt that the vitality of the plantar skin was inadequate to allow resection of an ellipse of skin as originally described by Fowler. Kates' procedure (Fig. 22.4) would have had a lesser corrective effect on the toe hammering and Lipscomb's proximal phalangeal excision plus condylectomy (Fig. 22.5) would have left the second metatarsal long.

4. The majority of patients are pleased with the early results of their surgery. They generally walk better and often are able to wear normal shoes for the first time in many years. Problems do arise, however, with time. In particular, patients may complain of progressive malalignment of the great toe, and the relative merits of hallux MTP fusion, joint arthroplasty and Keller's

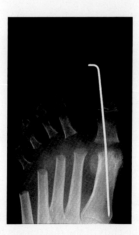

Fig. 22.3 Modified Fowler's procedure (Clayton)

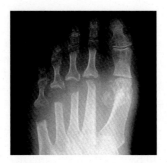

Fig. 22.4 Kates, Kessel, Kay procedure

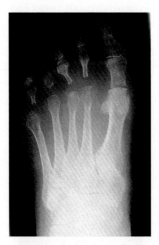

Fig. 22.5 Lipscomb's procedure

resection have not been well defined. Some patients complain of recurrent callosities across the plantar arch and a radiograph may reveal that the ends of the metatarsals have 'spiked'. A further local resection is often beneficial.

Key points

- Callosities form as the plantar fat pad is displaced distally.
- In rheumatoid arthritis the plantar skin will be atrophic.
- The surgeon must seek to provide a smooth metatarsal 'arc'.
- Partial phalangeal resection may be necessary if the toes are clawed.

Further reading

Fowler AW (1959) A method of forefoot reconstruction. Journal of Bone and Joint Surgery 41-B:507–13.

Karbowski A, Schwitalle M, Eckhardt A (1998) Arthroplasty of the forefoot in rheumatoid arthritis: long-term results after Clayton procedure. Acta Orthopaedica Belgica 64:401–5.

Kates A, Kessel L, Kay A (1967) Arthroplasty of the forefoot. Journal of Bone and Joint Surgery 49-B:552–7.

Lipscomb RR, Benson GM, Sones DA (1972) Resection of proximal phalanges and metatarsal condyles for deformities of the forefoot due to rheumatoid arthritis. Clinical Orthopedics 82:24–31.

Sharma DK, Roy N, Shenolikar A (2005) Weil osteotomy of lesser metatarsals for metatarsalgia: a clinical and radiological follow-up. The Foot 15:202–5.

Case 23

Patients generally present to the clinic with lesser deformity than that shown in Case 18. The radiograph opposite was taken of a 46-year-old secretary's foot (Fig. 23.1). She was simply troubled when she wore tight-fitting shoes, but had no pain at other times.

1. If the hallux valgus were to be addressed, what type of realignment should be performed?
2. Is there any place for a Keller's resection arthroplasty?
3. Can the displacement of the sesamoids shown be discounted?
4. Following surgery, when could the lady reasonably expect to be symptom free?

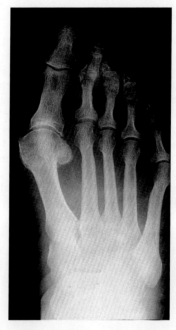

Fig. 23.1 Moderate hallux valgus

Surgery of hallux valgus

1. We believe that it is essential to maintain 'joint height' when performing a metatarsal osteotomy. Thus, if the first metatarsal is already short then any further shortening is ill advised. In the vast majority of individuals the intermetatarsal angle will be less than 15° and the deformity may be corrected by a distal osteotomy preserving length. This may be cut as a chevron, a scarf or Mitchell's displacement (Fig. 23.2) with a similar end result. Greater metatarsus varus is better treated by a Lapidus procedure (excision of the metatarso-cuneiform joint) or basal osteotomy (Fig. 23.3). An Akin phalangeal osteotomy may also be required to correct phalangeal angulation (Fig. 23.4).

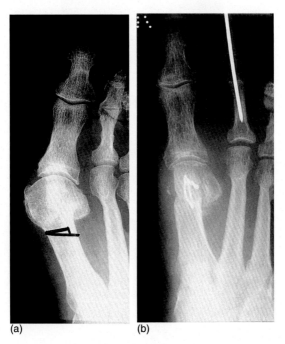

(a) (b)

Fig. 23.2 (a, b) Mitchell's osteotomy

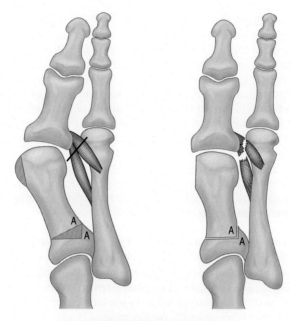

Fig. 23.3 Basal closing wedge osteotomy

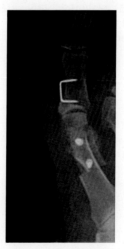

Fig. 23.4 Akin phalangeal osteotomy

2. The hallux is shortened and left 'floppy' after Keller's resection arthroplasty (removal of the proximal third of the proximal phalanx). It is not uncommon for the toe to 'cock up' and the loss of digit stability often leads to metatarsalgia because of disruption of the attachments of the plantar fascia and intrinsic muscles. The majority of young patients will not accept the inherent loss of 'push-off'. We would therefore only consider this procedure for inactive patients in late middle age, presenting with significant MTP joint arthritis.

3. The sesamoids, bound into flexor hallucis brevis, tend to retain their position as the hallux deviates medially. Since the central ridge on the underside of the metatarsal head may have flattened off as the medial sesamoid translocates, simply realigning the metatarsal may not be sufficient to restore the sesamoid to its natural position. A reefing of the medial joint capsule and sesamoidal ligament is usually required.

4. Most patients will be pleased with the results of corrective surgery provided that first metatarsal length is preserved. Union of any osteotomy will take a minimum of 6 weeks and often takes up to 12. We recommend immobilization of the foot in a fibreglass sabot cast for 6 weeks even if fixation is secure (Fig. 23.5). Malunion of the osteotomy is then less likely and we find that patients are more comfortable and in consequence generally more mobile.

Evidence

Evidence from 14 randomized trials suggests that chevron osteotomy is beneficial in the treatment of hallux valgus compared to orthoses or no treatment. When types of osteotomies were compared, no technique was shown to be superior to any other. It was notable that the numbers of participants in some trials remaining dissatisfied at follow-up were consistently high (25–33%), even when the hallux valgus angle and pain had improved.

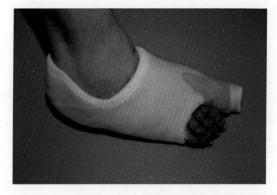

Fig. 23.5 Fibreglass sabot cast

Key points

- Shortening of the first metatarsal should be avoided.
- An attempt should be made to restore the sesamoids to their position below the metatarsal head.
- Long-term results of surgery are generally good.

Further reading

Ferrari J, Higgins JPT, Prior TD (2007) Interventions for treating hallux valgus (abductovalgus) and bunions. Cochrane Database of Systematic Reviews 2007, Issue 4. www.cochrane.org/reviews

Fokter SK, Podobnik J, Vengust V (1999) Late results of modified Mitchell procedure for the treatment of hallux valgus. Foot and Ankle International 20:296–300.

Judge MS, LaPointe S, Yu GV, Shook JE, Taylor RP (1999) The effect of hallux abducto-valgus surgery on the sesamoid apparatus position. Journal of the American Podiatric Medicine Association 89:551–9.

Pinney SJ, Song KR, Chou LB (2006) Surgical treatment of severe hallux valgus: the state of practice among academic foot and ankle surgeons. Foot and Ankle International 27:1024–9.

Trnka HJ, Zembsch A, Easley ME, Salzer M, Ritschl P, Myerson MS (2000) The chevron osteotomy for correction of hallux valgus. Comparison of findings after two and five years of follow-up. Journal of Bone and Joint Surgery 82-A:1373–8.

Zembsch A, Trnka HJ, Ritschl P (2000) Correction of hallux valgus. Metatarsal osteotomy versus excision arthroplasty. Clinical Orthopedics 376:183–94.

Section 4

Dermatology

Case 24

This 50-year-old woman presents with patchy loss of pigment over her feet and hands (Figs 24.1, 24.2).

1. What is the most likely cause of hypopigmentation of the feet and hands?
2. Are there any underlying diseases associated with hypopigmentation?
3. What other conditions may lead to loss of skin pigment and why is it a cause for concern in some countries?
4. What precautions should this lady be aware of?
5. Can it be treated?

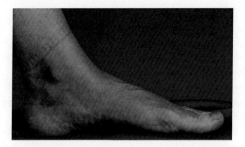

Fig. 24.1 Loss of skin pigment sole of left foot

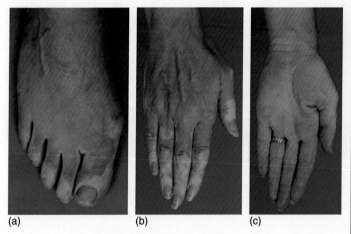

(a)   (b)   (c)

Fig. 24.2 Loss of skin pigment: (a) dorum of toes, (b) fingers and (c) left palm

Vitiligo

1. Vitiligo. It is a common acquired idiopathic disorder which displays well-defined irregular white areas (hypopigmentation). Lesions are often symmetrical.
2. The cause is thought to be autoimmune disease with antimelanocyte antibodies. Organ-specific autoimmune diseases such as Hashimoto's thyroiditis, Addison's hypoadrenalism, pernicious anaemia and diabetes are associated with vitiligo. Melanocytes are absent from the white lesions on histology.
3. Albinism and phenylketonuria cause generalized hypopigmentation whereas leprosy, tinea versicolor and lichen sclerosis result in patchy loss of skin pigment. Vitiligo can be mistaken for the depigmented patches of Hansen's disease (leprosy) and sufferers often become social outcasts.
4. The vitiliginous areas become easily sunburned and high factor sunscreen is required in the summer months.
5. Treatment can be unsatisfactory. Re-pigmentation can be achieved with exposure to long-wave ultraviolet light (UVA) together with psoralen (PUVA). Recent evidence shows that narrow band UVA (NB-UVA) is more effective than PUVA. The application of potent steroids can also induce re-pigmentation. Sunscreens reduce tanning of the pigmented skin and therefore reduce the contrast in skin tones. Cosmetic cover-up and self-tanning preparations can also be used.

Evidence

A systematic review of 19 RCTs revealed that potent topical steroids resulted in better repigmentation than placebo and they were also better than oral psoralens plus sunlight in another study. Two studies suggested that topical calcipotriol enhanced repigmentation rates from PUVAsol and PUVA when compared with placebo.

Key points

- Vitiligo is a common acquired disorder that displays well-defined irregular hypopigmentation.
- The cause is thought to be autoimmune disease with antimelanocyte antibodies.
- Vitiliginous areas become easily sunburned.
- Re-pigmentation can be achieved with exposure to long-wave ultraviolet light (UVA) together with psoralen (PUVA).

Further reading

Lim HW, Hexsel CL (2007) Vitiligo: to treat or not to treat. Archives of Dermatology 143:643-6.

Whitton ME, Ashcroft DM, Barrett CW, Gonzalez U (2006) Interventions for vitiligo. Cochrane Database of Systematic Reviews, Issue 1.

Yones S, Palmer R, Garibaldinos T, Hawk J (2007) Randomized double-blind trial of treatment of vitiligo: efficacy of psoralen-UV-A therapy vs narrowband-UV-B therapy. Archives of Dermatology 143:578-84.

Case 25

This 65-year-old man has discolouration of the skin over his lower leg and medial ankle (Fig. 25.1). He has been troubled by a recurrent ulcer in this area (Fig. 25.2).

1. What is the underlying pathology?
2. Explain the cause of the discolouration seen.
3. What management is appropriate?

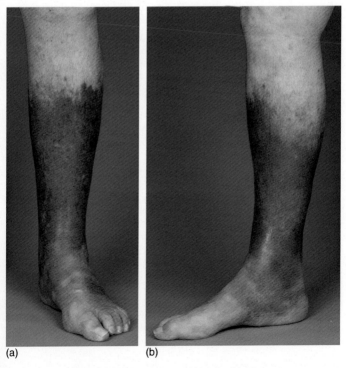

(a) (b)

Fig. 25.1 Skin discolouration: (a) left leg, (b) right leg

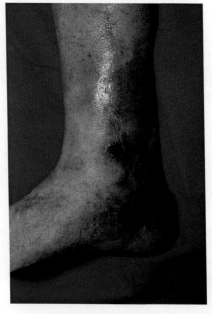

Fig. 25.2 Leg ulceration

Venous ulceration

1. Varicose eczema/ulceration (gravitational eczema) presents in elderly patients with venous hypertension. Incompetence of the deep venous valves allows reflux of blood that dilates the superficial veins. In consequence, there is a rise in capillary hydrostatic pressure and permeability that interferes with the diffusion of nutrients, which in turn leads to tissue necrosis. Fibrin is deposited as a pericapillary cuff around the ankle. This is termed lipodermatosclerosis.

2. The extensive discolouration seen in the 'gaiter region' of the leg is due to melanin deposition secondary to the chronic inflammation. Smaller areas of brown haemosiderin deposit (from extravasated red cells), telangiectasia and atrophie blanche (Fig. 25.3) can also occur.

3. Minor trauma to atrophic, eczematous skin often leads to ulceration and the essence of treatment is to reduce venous hypertension with the use of elevation and compression bandaging. Clearly this would be dangerous in the presence of arterial insufficiency and before any treatment is started, the patient's circulation should be assessed by Doppler scanning.

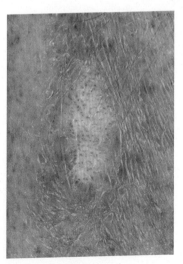

Fig. 25.3 Atrophy blanche

Blood pressure, heart rate and body mass index should also be measured and diabetes excluded. Once therapy starts, it is necessary to encourage walking and discourage prolonged standing to try and reduce stasis using the leg 'muscle pump'. Ulcer healing will be a slow, protracted process and probably require a regular application of dressings to the wound and oral therapies, including courses of diuretics and antibiotics.

Evidence

A systematic review for the Cochrane Library has shown no evidence of additional benefit associated with wound dressings, other than simple dressings, when used beneath compression bandaging. The conclusion was that inexpensive, simple non-adherent dressings should be used beneath compression therapy unless other factors, such as patient preference, take precedence.

Key points

- Arterial insufficiency should be excluded.
- Venous insufficiency is characterized by discolouration and varicose eczema on the lower leg.
- Ulcers follow minor trauma.
- Venous ulcer healing is protracted.

Further reading

Anderson I (2006) Aetiology, assessment and management of leg ulcers. Wound Essentials 1:20–38.

Moffat C (2001) Leg ulcers. In: Murray S (ed) Vascular disease: nursing and management. London: Whurr, 200–37.

Nelson EA, Bell-Syer SEM, Cullum NA (2000) Compression for preventing recurrence of venous ulcers. Cochrane Database of Systematic Reviews 2000, Issue 4.

Palfreyman SJ, Nelson EA, Lochiel R, Michaels JA (2006) Dressings for healing venous leg ulcers. Cochrane Database of Systematic Reviews 2006, Issue 3.

Case 26

A middle-aged woman presents with a persistent, red scaly rash on the outer aspect of her foot (Fig. 26.1). As can be seen in the figure, there are yellow pustules present. She has similar lesions on the palms of her hands that have been present for a considerable time. She is a smoker.

Younger patients often also present with similar erythematous lesions. The lesion shown in Figure 26.2 occurred in a young boy who was keen on sport and frequently wore training shoes.

1. Give the diagnosis for the first condition.
2. What is responsible for the erythematous lesion in the second condition?
3. What treatment would be appropriate in both instances?

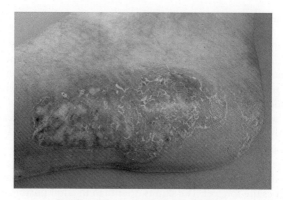

Fig. 26.1 Skin lesion on lateral border of foot

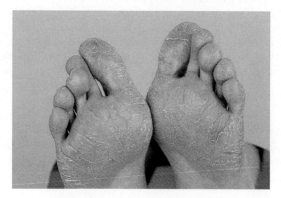

Fig. 26.2 Erythematous lesion of both feet

Plantar pustulosis/dermatosis

1. Palmoplantar pustulosis is a localized form of psoriasis which is confined to the palms and soles of middle-aged patients who invariably smoke. It frequently occurs without evidence of psoriasis elsewhere. It is characterized by sterile yellowish-white pustules that desiccate to leave discrete yellow-to-brown coloured stains. The surrounding skin is inflamed and scaly. Typically plantar pustulosis is seen along the medial longitudinal arches of the feet.

2. Juvenile plantar dermatosis is a scaly, glazed, fissured area of erythema seen on the weight-bearing areas of the feet, mainly across the forefeet. The skin is drier than in adult pustulosis and the condition is considered to be dermatitis from contact with synthetic materials.

3. Plantar pustulosis follows a protracted course and is often resistant to treatments such as coal tar, dithranol and steroids, although potent steroids and ultraviolet radiation may be beneficial. Treatment of the juvenile condition is easier, as often the children will be found wearing socks and shoes made from synthetic materials. They should try using an emollient cream such as Unguentum Merck and wear leather shoes if possible.

Key points

- Plantar pustulosis is a form of psoriasis seen on the feet.
- Juvenile plantar dermatosis is a contact dermatitis caused by synthetic footwear.
- Erythematous lesions are managed with steroids and emollients.

Further reading

Graham R (1989) Palmo-plantar pustulosis. Practitioner 233:1428–39.

Layton AM, Sheehan-Dare RA, Cunliffe WJ (1990) A double-blind placebo-controlled trial of topical PUVA in persistent palmoplantar pustulosis. British Journal of Dermatology 123 (s37):44–5.

Shackelford KE, Belsito DV (2002) The etiology of allergic-appearing foot dermatitis: a 5-year retrospective study. Journal of the American Academy of Dermatology 47(5):715–21.

This male patient worked in the mines for many years. He is now 74 years old and regularly attends for podiatric care of his toenails. On examination, all his toenails are thickened and discoloured (Fig. 27.1). He also has macerated skin between his fourth and fifth toes and there is a red scaly patch on the side of his right foot (Fig. 27.2).

1. Why is the condition of this ex-miner's toenails related to his previous work?
2. In more equivocal cases how should diagnosis be confirmed?
3. Is the condition of the nails associated with the scaly patch on the right foot (see Fig. 27.2)?
4. Do the nails and skin condition require treatment and if so, with what?

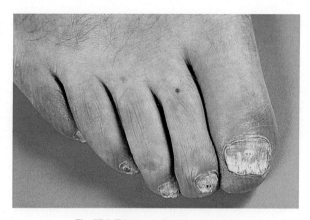

Fig. 27.1 Thickened, discoloured toenails

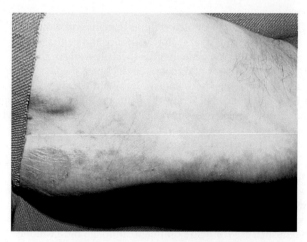

Fig. 27.2 Scaly patch on lateral border of right foot

Fungal foot infections

1. This man has a fungal infection of his nails (onychomycosis, tinea unguium). This condition used to be an occupational hazard of miners who shared communal bathing facilities. Fungal nail infections are caused by dermatophytes which digest keratin by producing enzymes. There are three genera of dermatophytes: *Microsporum*, *Trichophyton* and *Epidermophyton*. *Trichophyton rubrum* is the most common species of dermatophyte to infect the nails. The nail plate becomes thickened, separated from the nail bed, discoloured, brittle and develops a honeycombed structure. The fungus affects one or more nails but rarely all of them; this man being an exception to the rule. The condition is more common with increasing age.

2. In more equivocal cases, diagnosis can be confirmed by the finding of hyphae on microscopy. To identify a specific dermatophyte, the fungus must be cultured.

3. The scaly patch is athlete's foot (ringworm, tinea pedis), which is also caused by a superficial fungal infection similar to that seen in Figure 27.1.

4. This man was not troubled with his toenails and did not require treatment other than reassurance and palliative nail care. However, younger patients, especially women, can be more self-conscious of discoloured thickened toenails and are more likely to request treatment. Terbinafine (Lamisil) is an oral fungicidal which is now the mainstay of therapy for fungal nails, superseding griseofulvin, although amorolfine (Loceryl) is a nail lacquer that has some effect. Treatment should be continued for a full 3 months to eradicate the infection.

   Skin infection is more likely to respond to topical antifungal applications. In the first instance, patients should be given advice to dry their feet well after bathing, particularly between their toes. The use of astringents will reduce the moisture content of the skin and therefore the risk of infection. A topical agent such as Whitfield's ointment, although old-fashioned, is still useful but has been largely superseded by drugs of the azole (clotrimazole – Canesten, miconazole – Daktarin) and allylamine (terbinafine – Lamisil) groups.

Evidence

A systematic review of 67 RCTs shows convincing evidence that fungal skin infections are effectively managed by over-the-counter topical antifungal creams, lotions and gels. Terbinafine is the most effective topical agent.

There is some evidence that topical treatments (ciclopiroxolamine and butenafine) are effective for dermatophyte infections of the toenails but they need to be applied daily for at least 1 year.

Key points

- Fungal infections of the skin and toenails are common, affecting about 10% of the population.
- They are caused by dermatophyte infections.
- Skin and toenail infections are often found together.
- Infection of the skin requires advice and astringents or, if persistent, azoles or allylamines.

Further reading

Crawford F, Hollis S (1999) Topical treatments for fungal infections of the skin and nails of the foot. Cochrane Database of Systematic Reviews, Issue 3.

Gentles JC, Evans EGV (1973) Foot infections in swimming baths. British Medical Journal 3(5874):260–2.

Hart R, Bell-Syer SE, Crawford F, Torgerson D, Young P, Russell IT (1999) Systematic review of topical treatments for fungal infections of the skin and nails of the feet. British Medical Journal 319:79–82.

Roberts DT, Taylor WD, Boyle J (2003) Guidelines for treatment of onychomycosis. British Journal of Dermatology 148(3):402–10.

Case 28

A young student is troubled with a painful ingrowing toenail. His trouble first began when he cut down the side of his nail. As can be seen in Figure 28.1, his toe is infected and there is hypergranulation tissue present. He has had three courses of flucloxacillin. Each course brought about resolution of his infection but only for a few weeks.

1. Two distinct types of ingrowing toenail are recognized. Can you name them and what type does this young man have?
2. Why do the antibiotics only have a short-term effect?
3. Surgically, how is this painful toenail condition best treated?

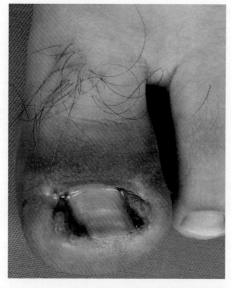

Fig. 28.1 Infected ingrowing toenail with hypergranulation tissue

Ingrowing toenails

1. Ingrowing toenails are a painful condition in which the nail edge penetrates the nail fold. There are two main causes. Ingrowth may be caused by a splinter of nail penetrating the nail sulcus (onychocryptosis), as presented on the previous page. This is more likely to occur if the nail plate is thin and broad, and is often accompanied by secondary infection and hypergranulation tissue. This type of nail problem is seen more often in young adult men and may be precipitated by poor nail cutting. Figure 28.2 shows an onychocryptosis with the spike of nail growing distally out of the end of the toe.

   In older women, where footwear may be a contributory factor, ingrowing toenails are caused by an increased transverse curvature of the nail (involuted or incurvature of the nail: Fig. 28.3). They are less likely to become infected but painful keratosis may develop in the nail folds. Poor management of these inwardly curved nails can lead to a spike of the involuted nail penetrating the skin as in onychocryptosis above.

2. Treatment of onychocryptosis with antibiotics resolves the immediate problem of infection but only temporarily, as the complaint soon recurs unless the offending portion of nail

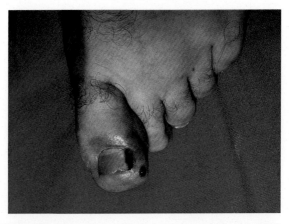

Fig. 28.2 Severe onychocryptosis with spike penetrating the end of the toe

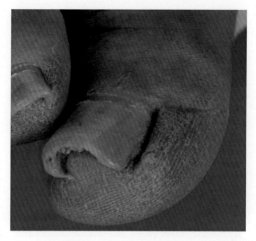

Fig. 28.3 Involution (incurvature) of the nail

is removed. Removal of the nail splinter and simultaneous narrowing will bring about a more satisfactory outcome. Removal of the entire nail is considered when the curvature of the toenail is too great or excessively thick (onychauxis or onychogryposis) and if fungal infection of the nail plate is present (onychomycosis).

3. Evidence shows that removal of part or the entire nail with phenolization is better than surgical excision alone (Zadik's or Winograd's procedures). Both Zadik's (total excision) and Winograd's (wedge excision) necessitate an extensive approach to completely expose the germinal matrix and are generally more painful for the patient postoperatively. There is a higher risk of regrowth of spikes of nail and thus failure of these procedures (Fig. 28.4).

The main benefit of phenol application is the reduced need for further operation because of recurrent nail growth; however, there is also less postoperative pain and bleeding. Furthermore, simple removal of the nail with phenolization is not precluded by the presence of infection and does not require skin suture. On the downside, it should be remembered that phenol is

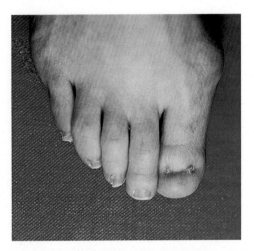

Fig. 28.4 Regrowth of nail spikes following Zadik's procedure

caustic and should be handled with extreme care. Phenol is also damaging to the wound tissues and may give rise to prolonged wound healing, increasing the risk of postoperative infection. These disadvantages are greatly outweighed by the advantages listed above.

Clinical tip

Apply an exsanguinating tourniquet (Esmarch bandage) around the toe. Identify the portion of nail to be removed. Separate this portion of nail plate from the nail bed and split the nail with a sharp chisel blade (Fig. 28.5a, b). Use forceps to gain a firm hold on the portion of nail and gently rotate towards the centre of the toe. Ensure that the nail matrix has been removed intact. Then, having applied Vaseline along the skin margin to protect it, apply minimum 80% strength phenol to the germinal matrix with a fine cotton bud and rub in well (Fig. 28.5c). Apply for a minimum of 3 minutes, then irrigate the nail fold with alcohol or saline solution. Dress the toe firstly with paraffin tulle gauze, then gauze swabs and secure with a tubular bandage.

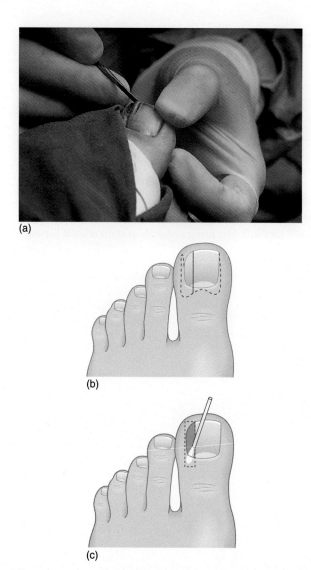

Fig. 28.5 (a, b) Removal of a lateral section of toenail. (c) Phenolization of germinal matrix

Evidence

Evidence from one systematic review for the Cochrane Library shows that removal of part or the entire nail with phenolization is better than surgical excision alone (Zadik's or Winograd's procedures).

One randomized controlled trial and one case control study show that podiatrists are more effective than surgeons at performing toenail surgery.

Key points

- Ingrowing toenails differ in aetiology in young and old patients.
- Antibiotics will only bring about short-term relief if the nail margin is not removed.
- Phenolization of the nail matrix is recommended after removal of the toenail.

Further reading

Gerritsma-Bleeker CL, Klaase JM, Geelkerken RH, Hermans J, van Det RJ (2002) Partial matrix excision or segmental phenolisation for ingrowing toenails. Archives of Surgery 137:320–5.

Laxton C (1995) Clinical audit of forefoot surgery performed by registered medical practitioners and podiatrists. Journal of Public Health Medicine 17:311–17.

Rounding C, Bloomfield S (2003) Surgical treatments for ingrowing toenails. Cochrane database of Systematic Reviews, Issue 1.

Shaath N, Shea J, Whiteman I, Zarugh A (2005) A prospective randomised comparison of Zadik procedure and chemical ablation in the treatment of ingrown toenails. Foot and Ankle International 26:401–5.

Thomson C, Paterson-Brown S, Russell IT (2002) A clinical and economic evaluation of toenail surgery performed by podiatrists in the community and surgeons in the hospital setting: a randomised controlled trial. www.show.NHS.uk/cso/.

Case 29

This is a common skin lesion that has appeared suddenly on the sole of this young swimmer's foot (Fig. 29.1). It has been present for about 6 weeks and appears to be getting larger. The boy's mother is demanding treatment.

1. Name this skin lesion.
2. Briefly describe the pathology of this lesion.
3. Which group of patients is at greater risk of this skin condition?
4. Should this mother's demands be met and, if so, what treatment is advocated?

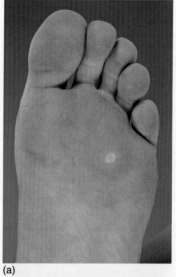

(a)

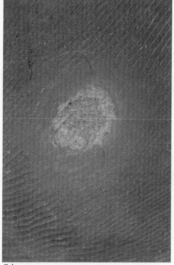

(b)

Fig. 29.1 (a, b) Lesion on the sole

Dermatology

Plantar warts

1. Plantar warts (verrucae) are common benign cutaneous
   tumours caused by infection of epidermal cells with human
   papilloma virus (HPV). Over 60 subtypes of DNA have been
   identified and HPV I, II and III are associated with plantar
   warts. They are seen in children and adolescents on the soles of
   the feet, where pressure causes them to grow into the dermis.
   Verrucae are more common in swimmers. The non-slip pool
   surfaces may macerate the skin, aiding inoculation of any free
   virus material. On the soles of the feet they can be difficult to
   distinguish from keratoses (corns) (Table 29.1).
2. The prickle cell layer of the epidermis becomes thickened
   and hyperkeratotic. Keratinocytes in the granular layer are
   vacuolated from infection with the wart virus.
3. Immunosuppressed individuals such as those with organ
   transplants are susceptible to viral warts. Mosaic warts are
   plaques on the soles that comprise multiple individual warts
   (Fig. 29.2). These are indicative of poor natural resistance
   to infection and present a difficult challenge. Figure 29.3
   shows large mosaic warts on the soles of the feet in a
   patient undergoing ciclosporin therapy 5 years after a heart
   transplant.

   Warts generally resolve spontaneously within 6 months in
   children. However, in adults they can persist for longer and
   sometimes for many years. As HPV is indirectly associated
   with epithelial malignancy (cervical cancer), there is a school

Table 29.1 Differentiation between a wart and a keratosis

Observation	Wart	Keratosis
After removal of overlying callus	Punctate spots (thrombosed capillaries), bleeding points	Skin concavity
Skin striae	Diverge from the lesion	Do not diverge
Site	Any site	Always weight-bearing site
Effect of lateral compression (pinching)	Very painful	Not painful

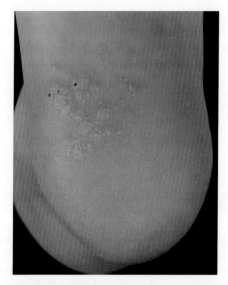

Fig. 29.2 Mosaic lesion

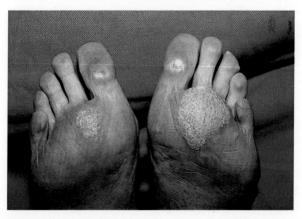

Fig. 29.3 Large mosaic warts on the soles of the feet in a patient undergoing ciclosporin therapy 5 years after a heart transplant

of thought that suggests that there is a value in allowing the child's immune system to be sensitized to the virus and therefore confer future immunity. The introduction of HPV vaccine for girls in the UK may result in a reduced incidence of warts in the future. As a rule of thumb, if plantar warts are painful, spreading, increasing in size or interfering with usual activities, then treatment is probably indicated. As this boy's lesion appears to be getting larger, then treatment should be considered.

There are a number of treatment options, none of which guarantees any form of success. The use of caustics and keratolytics has to be repeated at weekly intervals on several occasions and necessitates keeping the foot dry. There is evidence to support the use of 'duct' tape. It is suggested that by occluding the wart, the tape activates the immune system. Cryotherapy with either nitrous oxide or liquid nitrogen is a more painful but potentially more convenient alternative. Homeopathic remedies such as Thuja and Kalanchoe are less harmful options which the patient may administer themselves but claims as to their efficacy remain anecdotal at this time.

Occasionally, antiviral therapy such as intralesional bleomycin or immunotherapy such as dinitrochlorobenzene (DNCB) or diphencyprone may be indicated for recalcitrant lesions in adults.

Evidence

A systematic review of RCTs found that simple topical treatments containing salicylic acid were better than placebo. Two trials compared cryotherapy with salicylic acid and one compared duct tape with cryotherapy but there was no significant difference in efficacy. However, duct tape therapy is less expensive and has fewer adverse effects than cryotherapy.

Advice for patients (after Watkins)

- Do not attempt to pick or cut warts out.
- Avoid going barefoot in public areas.
- Cover affected areas with waterproof plasters or 'verruca socks'.
- If lesions are speading or getting bigger, seek medical help.

Key points

- Warts are common on the soles of the feet, particularly in children.
- Treatments include keratolytics and cryotherapy.
- Surface occlusion (e.g. verruca socks) will prevent 'contact' spread.

Further reading

Bunney M (1983) Viral warts. Edinburgh: Churchill Livingstone.

Focht DR, Spicer C, Fairchok MP (2002) The efficacy of duct tape vs cryotherapy in the treatment of verruca vulgaris (the common wart). Archives of Paediatrics and Adolescent Medicine 156(10):971–4.

Gibbs S, Harvey I. Topical treatments for cutaneous warts. Cochrane Database of Systematic Reviews 2001, Issue 2.

Watkins P (2006) Identifying and treating plantar warts. Nursing Standard 20(42):50–4.

Case 30

An athletic 20-year-old male student presents with a long-standing problem affecting both his feet (Fig. 30.1). His GP had never seen this problem before and so referred the student to a dermatology clinic.

1. Give the diagnosis.
2. Which organism is responsible?
3. Why are athletes more susceptible?
4. What is the treatment?

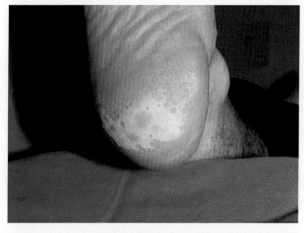

Fig. 30.1 Skin lesion on heel

Pitted keratolysis

1. Pitted keratolysis is a micrococcal bacterial infection caused by overgrowth of corynebacterium diphtheria commensals. Keratin is resorbed, producing pitting of the skin. The typical manifestation is of craterlike lesions on the plantar surfaces. These lesions appear on the pressure-bearing areas of the balls of the feet and heel pads where the keratin is more abundant.

2. Micrococci proliferate in moist conditions and patients with this complaint often sweat profusely (hyperhidrosis) and may wear occlusive footwear. There is usually an accompanying malodour.

3. Athletes are more susceptible because of increased moisture of the soles of the feet and formation of callouses.

4. The key to treatment is to deal with the hyperhidrosis. This student was treated successfully with formalin soaks. Other possible treatments include painting the skin with potassium permanganate or 2% erythromycin solution.

Key points

- Hyperhidrosis allows proliferation of skin pathogens.
- Pitted keratolysis is caused by a micrococcal infection.
- Hyperhidrosis is treated with astringents such as formalin or potassium permanganate soaks.

Further reading

Adams B (2002) Dermatologic disorders of the athlete. Sports Medicine 32(5):309–21.

Ramsey ML (1996) Pitted keratolysis: a common infection of active feet. The Physician and Sports Medicine 24(10).

Takama H, Tamada Y, Yano K, Nitta Y, Ikeya T (1997) Pitted keratolysis: clinical manifestations in 53 cases. British Journal of Dermatology 137:282–5.

Case 31

A middle-aged woman presents with chilblains and a history of painful, white fingers and toes on exposure to cold (Fig. 31.1).

1. What exactly is a chilblain?
2. With which connective tissue disorder is this condition associated?
3. How is the condition managed?

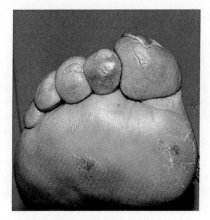

Fig. 31.1 Chilblains of the toes

Chilblains with Raynaud's phenomenon

1. Chilblains (perniosis) are a localized exaggerated response to cold, mostly affecting women and children, and commonly occurring on the fingers and toes. After exposure to cold there is prolonged constriction of the cutaneous arterioles and venules. The toes initially become red, hot and swollen because of a hyperaemic reaction and this is accompanied by intense itching. There follows a period of cyanosis and if the circulation does not improve, then ulcers form.

2. Chilblains are most commonly evident in patients with Raynaud's phenomenon. This condition is characterized by paroxysmal vasoconstriction of the digital vessels, causing the fingers and toes to turn white (due to ischaemia), become cyanotic (due to capillary dilatation with a stagnant blood flow) and then turn red (due to reactive hyperaemia). When Raynaud's is idiopathic it is termed a disease and when seen secondary to other conditions, it is termed a phenomenon. The disease is common. Ninety percent of patients are women and there is often a family history. Raynaud's phenomenon is associated with other connective tissue diseases, notably systemic sclerosis where a limited scleroderma may be associated with calcinosis, oesophageal involvement and telangiectasia – the CREST syndrome (Fig. 31.2).

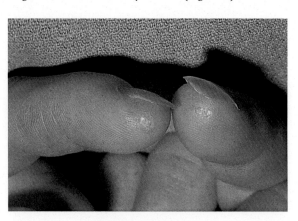

Fig. 31.2 Calcinosis cutis

Other causes of Raynaud's are:
- arterial occlusive conditions occurring in patients with atherosclerosis and Buerger's disease
- impaired vascular innervation occurring secondary to syringomyelia or paraplegia
- reflex vasoconstriction from occupational trauma, for example after prolonged typing or use of pneumatic tools
- bacterial toxins causing vasoconstriction
- increased blood viscosity.

3. Avoidance of cold is essential. Topical applications of 4% balsam of Peru are helpful but in many instances, where ulceration is recurrent, vasodilators such as the calcium channel blocker nifedipine may be required. Raynaud's is provoked by cold and therefore patients should be advised to keep their feet warm and avoid damp, cold conditions. In severe cases digital necrosis necessitates amputation.

Key points

- Chilblains are an exaggerated response to cold and are seen secondary to Raynaud's.
- Raynaud's is a vasoconstrictive disorder mainly affecting middle-aged women. It is associated with scleroderma in the CREST syndrome.
- Avoidance of cold is essential and vasodilators may be required.

Further reading

Dowd PM (1986) Nifedipine in the treatment of chilblains. British Medical Journal 293:923–40.

Isenberg DA, Black C (1995) ABC of rheumatology: Raynaud's phenomenon, scleroderma and overlap syndromes. British Medical Journal 310:795–8.

Kanwar AJ, Ghosh S, Dhar S (1992) Chilblain lupus erythematosus and lupus pernio – the same entity. Dermatology 185:160.

Section 5

At-risk foot

Case 32

A 72-year-old lady presents to the clinic concerned that she was walking on the outside of her foot. Clinical examination shows that she has a chronically discharging leg sinus (Fig. 32.1). This had been diagnosed as a varicose ulcer. A radiograph showed evidence of bone destruction (Fig. 32.2).

1. What is the likely cause of the radiological appearances?
2. This lady was suffering from minimal pain yet her ankle progressively adopted a varus deformity. What description is applied to painless arthritis?
3. How would you investigate this lady and what treatment is appropriate?

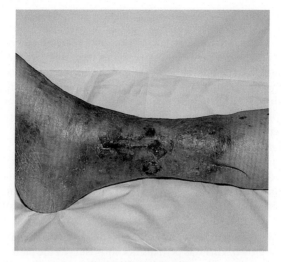

Fig. 32.1 Discharging sinus

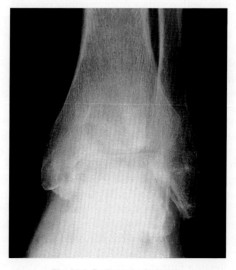

Fig. 32.2 Radiograph of left ankle

Septic arthritis

1. The radiograph shows cystic erosion of the tibial plafond, and the presence of peripheral osteophytes suggested that the joint destruction had developed over quite a long period. These appearances might have occurred in a patient with rheumatoid arthritis, but there were no other features of this condition. A copious discharge of purulent fluid made the diagnosis of a deep-seated infection straightforward.

2. Painless joint arthritis was described in patients with neurosyphilis by Charcot in 1858. The term 'Charcot joint' is now used as a generic term for joint destruction secondary to impaired sensation. The changes are most commonly seen in patients with diabetes mellitus although syphilis (tabes dorsalis), syringomyelia and congenital indifference to pain should also be considered.

3. A swab was sent for culture and sensitivity, but no organisms were grown. This was perhaps not surprising as the patient had been on several courses of antibiotics but both her erythrocyte sedimentation rate, at 86 mm/h, and C-reactive protein, at 350 mg/l, were greatly elevated.

   Drainage, with curettage of any necrotic material, is required to hasten healing. In this instance, however, such a procedure would almost certainly have destroyed any residual weight-bearing capacity that the patient had, and the end result would probably have been an amputation.

   It was no surprise when the microbiologist finally reported that the infection was due to tuberculosis. The patient was commenced on triple therapy (rifampicin, isoniazid and pyrazinamide) and the discharge diminished dramatically. Eighteen months after starting therapy the radiographic appearance was as shown in Figure 32.3. The patient had no pain and was walking in a surgical shoe with a heel flare, albeit using a stick outside. Although the degree of joint subluxation will almost certainly mean that she will need to wear a leg caliper in the future, this would clearly be preferable to either a joint fusion or amputation. A fusion would not only be technically difficult to achieve in the presence of such significant bone destruction, but it is unlikely that the lady would tolerate a further 6–8 weeks in a plaster cast.

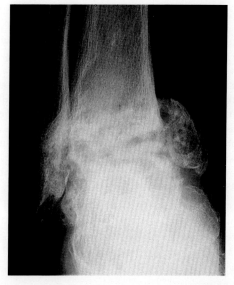

Fig. 32.3 Distal tibia and ankle after 18 months' chemotherapy

Key points

- Some form of neuropathy must be present in patients with a Charcot joint.
- All patients should be tested for diabetes mellitus.
- Consider tuberculosis as a cause of chronic sepsis.

Further reading

Dhillon MS, Nagi ON (2002) Tuberculosis of the foot and ankle. Clinical Orthopaedics and Related Research 398:107–13.

Laing P (2000) Surgical management of the Charcot foot. The Diabetic Foot 3:44–8.

Case 33

A 58-year-old male railway worker is referred by his GP with pain in his right foot. An X-ray of his foot had previously shown degenerative changes in the MTP joint.

The patient indicates that his pain arises in his great toe and extends into the dorsum of his foot. Pain occurs after walking for about 5–10 minutes. The pain becomes so intense that he has to stop and rest before the pain eases and he can walk once more. He is also troubled with cramps at night that frequently disturb his sleep. He is a heavy smoker.

On removing his shoes, there is an obvious pallor of his right foot (Fig. 33.1).

1. Which eponym is used to describe the test conducted in Figure 33.2 and what is the physiological principle behind this test?
2. What key features are observed (a) with the limbs elevated (Figs 33.2, 33.3) and (b) on dependency (Fig. 33.4)?
3. What is your diagnosis and what would be your pathway of care for this patient?

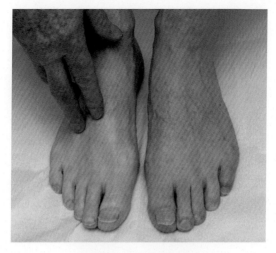

Fig. 33.1 Pallor of right foot

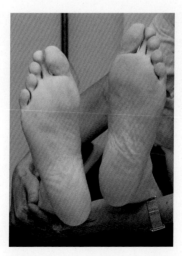

Fig. 33.2 Plantar aspect of feet with both limbs elevated (note the contrast between the right and left feet)

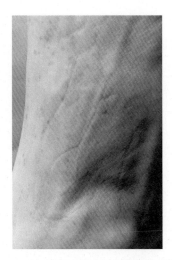

Fig. 33.3 Close-up of 'guttering' of veins of right foot, with limb elevated

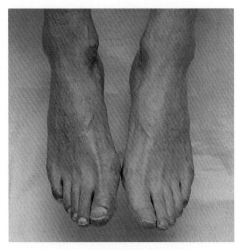

Fig. 33.4 Dependency of both limbs: note reactive hyperaemia in right foot

Critical limb ischaemia

1. This is Buerger's limb elevation test. Under normal circumstances sufficient arterial pressure should exist to maintain an adequate blood supply to the feet and toes even with the limb elevated. However, when there is arterial compromise, i.e. atherosclerosis, the arterial pressure is reduced and the foot is deprived of blood. To carry out this test, the patient should be laid flat and the legs elevated well above the level of the heart and subsequent observations recorded. The limbs should be kept elevated for about 3 minutes and the features observed. The legs are then lowered with the patient in a sitting position and observed for a further 3 minutes.

   This is a useful test to use in conjunction with measurement of the ankle brachial pressure indices when calcification of the arteries is suspected.

2. In the presence of significant disease a number of features can be observed.

   With the limbs elevated:
   • a rapid pallor of the right foot in comparison to the normal limb (see Fig. 33.2)
   • a rapid emptying of veins (guttering; see Fig. 33.3)
   • an absent or reduced capillary filling time.

   With the limbs dependent:
   • the rate of refilling of veins will be sluggish on the affected side
   • the time taken for the pallor to subside is also relevant and this time is increased on the right side
   • there is increased rubor (dusky red colouration) of the foot as a result of prolonged deprivation of oxygen, known as reactive hyperaemia (see Fig. 33.4). Compare the colour with that evident in Figure 33.1.

3. Critical limb ischaemia. This condition threatens life and limb. A suggested pathway of care is illustrated in Table 33.1.

   In this case, the patient was seen urgently by a vascular surgeon. Specialized investigations including Doppler scanning and a femoral angiogram revealed extensive atheroma in the femoral and iliac arteries. A cross-over graft was necessary from the right femoral artery but although, his peripheral arterial circulation improved to 60% of normal, he was unable to return to work.

Table 33.1 Pathway of care for critical limb ischaemia

Symptoms	Pathway
Intermittent claudication without ulceration	Encourage exercise to open up collateral vessels. Smoking cessation. Monitor.
Rest pain	Refer to vascular surgeon. Check blood pressure and cholesterol levels, with appropriate drug management if appropriate.
Ulceration/gangrene	Establish extent of atherosclerosis. Consider intervention such as grafting, bypass surgery or amputation.

Evidence

Lumbar sympathectomy is a minimally invasive procedure with a low complication rate. Three randomized controlled trials have failed to identify any objective benefits for lumbar sympathectomy. However, subjective improvements in symptoms for patients with highly symptomatic critical leg ischaemia have been consistently demonstrated in ten cohort studies, with sustained symptom improvements in approximately 60% of patients. Lumbar sympathectomy should be considered for symptomatic patients with critical leg ischaemia as an alternative to amputation in patients with otherwise viable limbs.

Key points

- Claudication and rest pains are an indication of significant peripheral arterial disease.
- Buerger's limb elevation is a quick, easy test that does not require expensive equipment.

- It is important to address other risk factors such as smoking, hyperlipidaemia and hypertension.
- Abstinence from tobacco products is the only way to prevent disease progression.

Further reading

Paraskevas KI, Liapis CD, Briana DD, Mikhailidis DP (2007) Thromboangiitis obliterans (Buerger's disease): searching for a therapeutic strategy. Angiology 58:75–84.

Sanni A, Hamid A (2005) Is sympathectomy of benefit in critical leg ischaemia not amenable to revascularisation? Best BETs. www.bestbets.org

Sasajima T, Kubo Y, Izumi Y, Inaba M, Goh K (1994) Plantar or dorsalis pedis artery bypass in Buerger's disease. Annals of Vascular Surgery 8:248–57.

Case 34

A 40-year-old holidaymaker is out walking through wet grass adjacent to a Scottish links golf course. He is aware of a sharp 'stab' on the top of his foot. Within minutes he is unable to bear weight and on removing his sock, he notices that his skin has been punctured (Fig. 34.1). Six hours later his entire leg is bruised and swollen up to the knee.

1. What is the likely predator?
2. What investigations are appropriate?
3. What should be his acute management?
4. Where may antivenom be obtained?

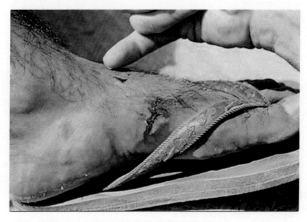

Fig. 34.1 Perforating wound

Snake bite

1. The adder (*Vipera berus* – Fig. 34.2) is the only indigenous venomous snake in the UK and snakebite is rare but still, as elsewhere in the world, potentially lethal. In the US the two main families of venomous snakes are the Crotalidae (pit vipers, including the rattlesnake, cottonmouth and copperhead) and the Elapidae (coral snakes).

   After a bite on the foot or ankle there is rapid peripheral swelling and a spreading inflammatory process (similar to cellulitis) will be evident. Haemorrhagic blebs develop at the site of the bite within 6–36 hours. Palpation of the groin will reveal regional lymphadenopathy and systemic effects are soon apparent. Generally the patient will become nauseous, and vomiting, diarrhoea, incontinence, vasoconstriction and pronounced tachycardia are common. Angio-oedema with swelling of the face and tongue leading to airway obstruction and hypotension may be fatal.

2. Investigations should include examination of a blood film and measurement of serum creatine kinase (indicative of muscle necrolysis). Bleeding is rare but may be secondary to thrombocytopenia. An electrocardiograph will exclude any myocardial ischaemia.

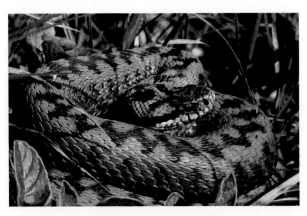

Fig. 34.2 *Vipera berus* (adder)

3. Supportive therapy is required from the moment of presentation. This should include immobilization of the affected leg in a splint and immediate transfer to hospital. If the snake has been killed then it should be identified on site or taken to the hospital. A stick longer than the snake's length is required to pick it up, to avoid any further envenomation. Pressure immobilization (by firm bandaging but not tourniquet) is particularly important for bites by snakes of the Elapidae family (coral snakes, kraits and mambas). Adequate analgesia should be prescribed and adrenaline (epinephrine) kept close by in case of anaphylaxis. Envenoming may be quite slow and the patient should be admitted to hospital for at least 24 hours.

4. Antivenom is obtained through the major hospital casualty departments sourced generally from a National Poisons Centre. Care should always be taken if antivenom is administered as this may also induce anaphylaxis.

Evidence

One randomized controlled trial from Sri Lanka showed that giving adrenaline with antivenom reduced the rate of adverse reactions. One Brazilian study showed no benefit of antihistamine drugs. No trials report on the role of corticosteroids.

Key points

- Venomous pit vipers have triangular heads, elliptic eyes, heat-sensing pits on the sides of their heads, a single row of ventral scales and rattles on the tail.
- Non-venomous pit vipers have rounded heads, spherical eyes, a double row of ventral scales and no rattle.
- Venomous elapids have short fangs, round pupils, a double row of subcaudal scales and red bands bordered by yellow or white as shown in Figure 34.3. A few non-venomous species in the US only are identified by the black band approximating to the red ('Red to yellow, kill a fellow. Red to black, venom lack').
- Pressurization will delay venom spread by collapsing small veins and lymphatics.

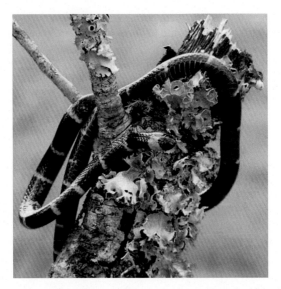

Fig. 34.3 *Micrurus fulvius fulvius* (Eastern coral snake). Photo by Michael Dye – *www.floridabackyardsnakes.com*

Further reading

Aurerback PS, Donner HJ, Weiss EA (1999) Snake and reptile bites. In: Field guide to wilderness medicine. St Louis: Mosby, 253–65.

Nuchpraryoon I, Garner P (1999) Interventions for preventing reactions to snake antivenom. Cochrane Database of Systematic Reviews, Issue 4.

Warrell DA (2005) Treatment of bites by adders and exotic venomous snakes. British Medical Journal 331:1244–7.

Case 35

This young nurse presented with a 12-week history of discolouration of her toenail (Fig. 35.1). She first became aware of the lesion when on a 'holiday in the sun'. According to the patient, the lesion has remained static in size since that time.

1. Why is the history of this lesion atypical?
2. What is your provisional diagnosis and which investigations should be carried out at initial consultation?
3. How are these lesions graded?
4. What do you do now?

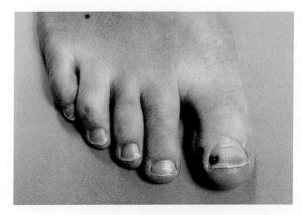

Fig. 35.1 Discolouration of toenail

Melanoma

1. This subungual nail lesion is atypical of trauma. Haematoma normally subside within a few weeks and therefore one would have expected the lesion to have faded. Given the duration and the appearance of the discolouration, further investigation is necessary.

2. It should be an immediate concern that the lesion is a malignant melanoma. Careful examination is required to detect the presence of satellite lesions, and the drainage lymph nodes in the popliteal fossa and groin should be examined for enlargement. Other diagnoses include pyogenic granuloma, onychomycosis, a subungual naevus and a subungual exostosis. A radiograph would immediately exclude the last diagnosis.

   Acral lentiginous melanomas make up 10% of UK melanoma cases. They are found on the soles of the feet (Fig. 35.2), the palms of the hands and under the nails. Subungual melanoma was first described by Hutchison in 1883.

3. Melanoma are locally staged according to how thick and deep the lesions are (Breslow grade) and clinically by regional spread (Clark classification) (Table 35.1).

4. If this lesion is shown to be a melanoma then immediate intervention has a bearing on the patient's survival rate. A diagnosis is required urgently. This girl went on to have her nail removed and an excisional biopsy performed within 2 days. The lesion was in fact blood. Treatment might otherwise have been as shown in Table 35.2.

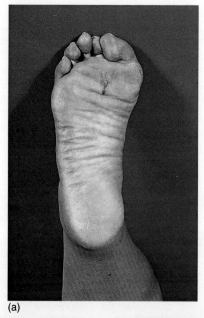

(a)

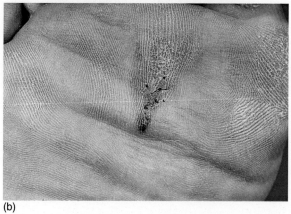

(b)

Fig. 35.2 Infiltrating melanoma on sole

Table 35.1 Staging and prognosis of malignant melanoma

	Thickness	Spread	Prognosis
Stage I	<1.5 mm	Upper dermis	Excellent
Stage II	1.5–4 mm	Deep layers of skin – not lymph nodes	May be cured – ? distant metastases
Stage III	>4 mm	Lymph node infiltration. Possible satellite lesions	Better survival if only to local nodes
Stage IV	>4 mm	Distant metastases	<5% 5-year survival

Table 35.2 Treatment recommendations for hand and foot melanomas

Microscopic Thickness of Primary Melanoma	Dorsum	Subungual	Acral Lentiginous
<1.5 mm	Excision with 1 cm margin*	Amputation of distal phalanx	Excision with 1 cm margin*
≥1.5 mm	Excision with 2 cm margin* plus sentinel lymph node biopsy†	Amputation of distal phalanx plus sentinel lymph node biopsy†	Excision with 2 cm margin* plus sentinel lymph node biopsy†

*Skin grafting may be necessary in some cases.
†Regional lymphadenectomy if sentinel node contains melanoma.
(reproduced with permission from Tseng (1997) Ann Surg 225(5):544–553)

Key points

- All pigmented subungual lesions should be viewed with suspicion
- Liaison with the local tumour centre is required before biopsy.
- Full-thickness excisional biopsy performed under local anaesthesia is the preferred biopsy technique.
- Shave biopsies are contraindicated as they do not allow assessment of melanoma depth.
- Acral lentiginous malignant melanoma are often diagnosed late and have a poor prognosis.

Further reading

Finlay RK, Driscoll DL, Blumenson LE, Karakousis CP (1994) Subungual melanoma: an eighteen year review. Surgery 116:96–100.

Gray RJ, Pockaj BA, Vega ML et al (2006) Diagnosis and treatment of malignant melanoma of the foot. Foot and Ankle International 27:696–705.

Tseng JF, Tanabe KK, Gadd MA et al (1997) Surgical management of primary cutaneous melanomas of the hands and feet. Annals of Surgery 225:544–50.

Case 36

A 75-year-old man presents with skin atrophy and potential ulcer formation under his first and fifth metatarsal heads. The medial hallux sesamoid was excised and a sliding fifth metatarsal osteotomy satisfactorily lessened the pressure on the skin laterally. Unfortunately, the short 1 cm lateral surgical incision would not heal.

1. What other diagnostic tests should be requested?
2. What options are there for further treatment?
3. If amputation is required, which would be most appropriate for this man?

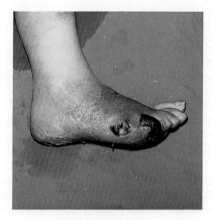

Fig. 36.1 Infected foot

Amputation

1. Clearly the fifth digit is gangrenous and there is significant infection spreading through the soft tissues of the forefoot. Untreated diabetes would be one's first thought, but in this instance there was no evidence of urinary glucose excretion and a random blood sugar was within normal limits (3–6 mmol/l). The patient's erythrocyte sedimentation rate was, however, elevated and a subsequent blood film revealed a proliferation of myeloblastic precursor cells compatible with an acute myeloid leukaemia.

   To establish whether the infection extended into the metatarsals, a radiograph was requested and peripheral vascularity was assessed by Doppler ultrasound scanning.

2. There was no radiographic evidence of osteomyelitis, but a rampant cellulitis developed despite intravenous antibiotic therapy. Since the average life expectancy for patients with acute myeloid leukaemia is less than 6 months, a below-knee amputation was selected as being the most likely method of producing a healed stump and a rapid restoration of mobility. A long posterior flap was cut to take advantage of the better perfusion of the posterior calf skin and facilitate stump healing.

3. A Syme's amputation (Fig. 36.2) was considered, but it was felt that if this were to fail, the patient might spend the majority of his remaining life in hospital. Although it would have been possible to stage the amputation, reducing the risk of spread of infection to the tibia, healing of a Syme's stump is entirely dependent on an adequate blood supply to the heel from the calcaneal branches of the posterior tibial artery. At stage one, the foot is removed leaving the tibial articular cartilage and malleoli, with the wounds closed in standard fashion over a suction drain. Antibiotics can then be instilled locally as a prophylaxis against spread of infection, although most surgeons simply administer these parenterally. At 6 weeks, the malleoli are trimmed through two short incisions and a temporary Syme's prosthesis may be fitted.

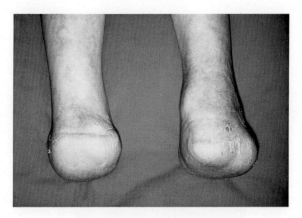

Fig. 36.2 Syme's amputation stumps

A simple fifth ray, a Lisfranc's (tarsometatarsal) or Chopart's (midtarsal) amputation, would have been doomed to failure because of the oedema and swelling of the dorsal foot skin. Similarly, both Boyd's calcaneotibial fusion and Pirogoff's calcaneal section/rotational amputation were discounted as being unnecessarily complicated in this instance. In any case, both the latter two procedures depend on fusion of the calcaneal remnant to the tibia and require at least 8 weeks' stump immobilization in plaster. In contrast, this patient was mobile on a custom prosthesis similar to that shown in Figure 36.3 within 1 month.

Key points

- Always check peripheral circulation and sensation before choosing the resection level.
- Seek the opinion of a second surgeon before proceeding.
- Beware of foot equinus following Lisfranc's amputation and equinovalgus after Chopart's amputation.
- A Syme's stump will allow direct end weightbearing.
- Staging a Syme's amputation may prevent the spread of sepsis.

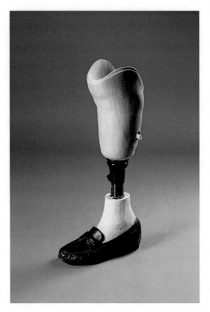

Fig 36.3 Custom below-knee prosthesis with solid ankle cushion heel

Further reading

Burgess EM, Romano RL, Zettl JH, Schrock RD (1971) Amputations of the leg for peripheral vascular insufficiency. Journal of Bone and Joint Surgery 53-A:874–90.

Frykberg RG, Abraham S, Tierney E, Hall J (2007) Syme amputation for limb salvage: early experience with 26 cases. Journal of Foot and Ankle Surgery 46:93–100.

Grady JF, Winters CL (2000) The Boyd amputation as a treatment for osteomyelitis of the foot. Journal of the American Podiatric Medicine Association 90:234–9.

Stone PA, Back MR, Armstrong PA (2005) Midfoot amputations expand limb salvage rates for diabetic foot infections. Annals of Vascular Surgery 19:805–11.

Case 37

A man presents with a painful ulcer on his big toe. His ankle brachial pressure index (ABPI) is 0.5. A radiograph of his distal phalanx reveals an underlying osteomyelitis (Fig. 37.1).

1. What is the ABPI?
2. How is it measured?
3. Is this an absolute test?
4. What does an ABPI of 0.5 indicate and how should this patient be managed?

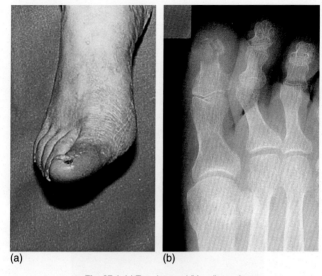

Fig. 37.1 (a) Toe ulcer and (b) radiograph

Ischaemic toe

1. The ABPI is a useful and easily performed clinical technique. It is a sensitive test for arterial insufficiency and provides quantitative information about the arterial supply to the foot.

2. The taking of the ABPI requires measurement of the systolic blood pressure at the arm and ankle. Both values may be obtained with a handheld Doppler ultrasound probe and sphygmomanometer (Fig. 37.2). Systolic pressure at the ankle should equal the central (brachial) pressure, although, in fact, owing to the decrease in calibre of distal vessels, the ankle systolic pressure is normally greater. The pressure index

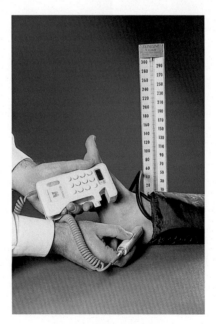

Fig. 37.2 ABPI measurement

is the ratio of ankle:brachial systolic pressure. Patients with significant atherosclerosis, exhibiting signs of claudication, will have a value of greater than 0.5 but less than 1. A value of less than 0.5 requires urgent vascular intervention (Table 37.1).

3. Although generally a sensitive and reliable measurement, false-positive values may occur if there is any arterial calcification (Mönckeberg's sclerosis), in diabetes and in the elderly. Although calcification of the arterial media will not obstruct blood flow, the vessels become less compressible and will lead to a falsely high ABPI. In these cases, attention should be paid to the quality of the Doppler wave form, which should be biphasic or triphasic. A monophasic wave form is indicative of arteriosclerosis. The ABPI can also be used in combination with a subjective evaluation of the circulation such as by Buerger's limb elevation test (see Fig. 33.2), in which the leg is raised and noted for pallor. On dependency, the return of colour should be brisk. Delayed filling, cyanosis or hyperaemia is indicative of ischaemia. For patients with diabetes mellitus with arterial calcification, the measurement of toe systolic pressures is recommended.

Table 37.1 ABPI values, interpretation and implications

ABPI value (x)		Interpretation	Implication
$x \geq 1.3$		Calcification of arteries	Attention required to Doppler wave form toe pressures and pole test
$1 \geq x < 1.3$		Normal	
$0.5 \geq x < 1$	Upper limit	Minor disease	Delayed wound healing
	Mid-range	Claudication	Significant, symptomatic disease
	Lower limit	Rest pain	Limb at risk from ulceration
$x < 0.5$		Critical limb ischaemia	Vascular surgery

4. The implication of an abnormal ABPI for this man is that his ulcer will not heal until the arterial supply has been improved. The lesion is complicated by underlying osteomyelitis evident in Figure 37.1b for which antibiotics will be ineffective because of the lack of a blood supply. He requires arteriography and probably amputation.

Key points

- The ABPI is a sensitive measure which is useful for quantifying arterial disease.
- Calcification of the arteries will result in a falsely high ABPI.
- Buerger's limb elevation test should be used to complement ABPI measurements.
- Ulcer healing will not take place until a blood supply has been re-established.

Further reading

Donnelly R, Emslie-Smith AM, Gardner ID, Morris AD (2000) Vascular complications of diabetes. British Medical Journal 320:1062–6.

Donnelly R, Hinwood D, London NJM (2000) Non-invasive methods of arterial and venous assessment. British Medical Journal 320:698–701.

Grasty MS (1999) Use of the hand-held Doppler to detect peripheral vascular disease. Diabetic Foot 2(suppl):18–21.

Vowden P (1999) Doppler ultrasound in the management of the diabetic foot. Diabetic Foot 2(suppl):16–17.

Case 38

A 54-year-old man was admitted to the trauma unit after his right great toe became swollen. He had no recollection of an injury. An X-ray did not show clear evidence of a lesion but a subsequent MRI revealed significant bone destruction (Fig. 38.1).

1. What are the differential diagnoses of this lesion?
2. Are there any specific attributes that would define a cartilaginous lesion?
3. What treatment is warranted?

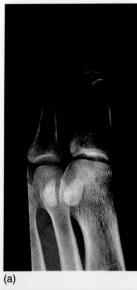

(a)

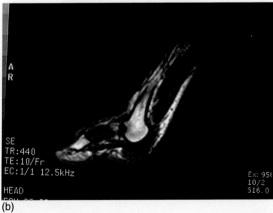

(b)

Fig. 38.1 (a) Radiograph and (b) sagittal T1-weighted MR image of right great toe

Chondrosarcoma of the great toe

1. The radiograph demonstrated very little but a well-defined lytic lesion was evident on the MR image shown. The most immediate concern would be that this was a metastatic deposit, but other possible diagnoses would be an intraosseous ganglion, benign tumour of tendon sheath or enchondroma. Multiple lesions would be pathognomonic of Ollier's disease or multiple enchondromatosis.

2. Microscopy of a biopsy from the lesion (Fig. 38.2) showed a cellular and lobulated tumour with islands of cartilage filling up the marrow spaces. The nuclei shown are large and both nucleoli and binucleate cells are not difficult to find. Even though there are no mitoses in the section, the cellularity and atypia of the cells make this lesion typical of a chondrosarcoma.

3. After a preliminary biopsy, it is necessary to excise any tumour mass completely, including the biopsy tract. In this instance amputation of the toe was required as, although the tumour was low grade, a wide excision would have left no viable tissue.

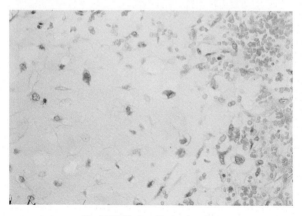

Fig. 38.2 Biopsy of lesion from toe

The patient was subsequently fitted with a total contact insole combined with a toe spacer to compensate for the amputation. It is not likely that any other treatment will be required in the future for this low-grade lesion and the patient's life expectancy should be normal.

Key points

- Malignant tumours are fairly common in the foot. Beware of melanoma in particular.
- Biopsy may spread a tumour and preclude definitive local resection. Therefore refer to a specialist unit before biopsy if the diagnosis is uncertain.
- Complete excision often necessitates amputation.
- Chemotherapy or radiotherapy may be required.

Further reading

Bovee JV, van der Heul RO, Taminiau AH, Hogendoorn PC (1999) Chondrosarcoma of the phalanx: a locally aggressive lesion with minimal metastatic potential: a report of 35 cases and a review of the literature. Cancer 86:1724–32.

Gajewski DA, Burnette JB, Murphey MD, Temple HT (2006) Differentiation clinical and radiographic features of enchondroma and secondary chondrosarcoma in the foot. Foot and Ankle International 27:240–4.

Case 39

A 60-year-old man is admitted to the medical ward on 2 January, having been found lying in a disused railway shed. It is noted that his toes are white in colour and somewhat insensitive. Unfortunately, over the next few days the appearance dramatically changes (Fig. 39.1).

1. What is the likely cause of this man's foot ischaemia?

2. What factors have led to the appearances found?

3. Is there an urgent need for surgical treatment and what operation would be appropriate?

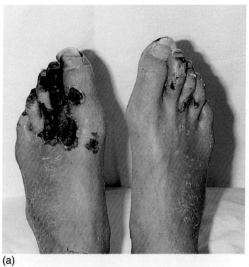

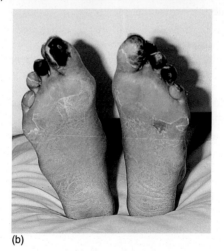

Fig. 39.1 Toe lesions

Frostbite

1. On arrival in casualty, the patient was found to have a temperature of 35.5°C and it was felt that he had probably been exposed to the elements for some time. Gradual warming soon brought his temperature up to a normal level and restored the colour to his toes, although they became slightly 'mottled'. The initial changes were at first felt to be caused by a generally poor peripheral circulation, but later skin blistering and necrosis were typical of frostbite.

2. The primary aetiological factor in this instance was a prolonged exposure to cold, causing reduced peripheral blood flow by vasoconstriction and increased plasma viscosity. The situation had not been improved by the patient's consumption of alcohol over the New Year, causing dehydration by diuresis. The patient was probably lying immobile for several hours and it was important to exclude a calf or foot compartment syndrome. Either would reduce venous drainage from the periphery and accentuate any ischaemia.

3. Gradually the area of ischaemic tissue demarcated. In areas where small superficial blisters were present, a black eschar formed. This separated off in places, leaving a raw area denuded of skin (as shown on the dorsum of the great toe in Figure 39.1a). Circumferential injury, however, necessitated amputation.

   Theoretically the digits would have spontaneously separated off by 'autoamputation', but this may take in excess of 3 months and it was considered preferable to excise the affected toes surgically as soon as the limitation of the ischaemia was apparent.

   Frostbite is a form of gangrene and it is therefore essential to ensure that patients are covered against tetanus. Antibiotic treatment is not required unless a spreading cellulitis develops.

1912

'I am just going outside and may be some time' – Lawrence 'Titus' Oates to Captain Robert Scott, Antarctica, March 1912. Oates had developed severe frostbite which prevented him from keeping pace with Scott, Bowers and Wilson on their return from the South Pole. He perished on his 32nd birthday.

Key points

- Frostbite should be suspected in patients with hypothermia.
- Check the patient's tetanus immunity.
- Muscle injury with rhabdomyolysis and neural injury may be present.

Further reading

Cauchy E, Marsigny B, Allamel G, Verhellen R, Chetaille E (2000) The value of technetium 99 scintigraphy in the prognosis of amputation in severe frostbite injuries of the extremities: a retrospective study of 92 severe frostbite injuries. Journal of Hand Surgery 25A:969–78.

Pulla RJ, Pickard LJ, Carnett TS (1994) Frostbite: an overview with case presentations. Journal of Foot and Ankle Surgery 33:53–63.

Case 40

A 55-year-old lady is referred as an emergency. She presents with a painful swollen foot. There is a wound on the sole with a spreading cellulitis apparent along the medial longitudinal arch (Fig. 40.1). She feels generally unwell, having flu-like symptoms.

1. Describe the clinical features apparent in Figure 40.1.
2. This lady does not have the flu but why did she present with these symptoms?
3. Outline the further investigations which were required in this instance.
4. Discuss your immediate management of this patient.
5. What factors have predisposed to this foot condition and how does this influence your management?

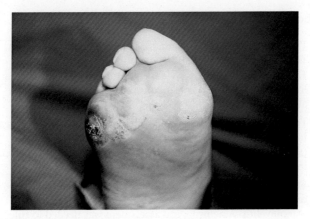

Fig. 40.1 Plantar aspect of foot

Subcutaneous infection

1. The clinical features apparent are cellulitis and lymphangitis. There is a cavity of pus underlying the subcutaneous tissue. The infection is spreading via the lymph vessels in the medial longitudinal arch and is seen 'tracking'. Tissue destruction is also evident.

2. This patient has early signs of septicaemia. Bacteria have spread into the bloodstream (bacteraemia) and are multiplying (septicaemia). Popliteal and inguinal lymph nodes are tender, indicating lymphadenitis.

3. Bacteriological culture identified the precise causative micro-organism as *Streptococcus pyogenes* and X-rays excluded osteomyelitis. A neurological assessment was needed to rule out a neuropathy and a vascular assessment to quantify tissue perfusion. Later, foot pressure assessment was carried out to assess plantar pressure distribution.

4. Immediate treatment involved drainage of the lesion (Fig. 40.2). The patient was also given strict advice to rest and prescribed erythromycin 500 mg qds for the spreading infection (Table 40.1).

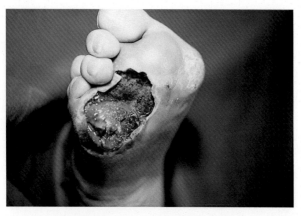

Fig. 40.2 Debridement and drainage of the lesion

Table 40.1 A guide to typical antibiotic therapy for subcutaneous infection

Organism	Description therapy	Antimicrobial therapy: first-line
Staphylococcus aureus	Abcesses, yellow pus	Flucloxacillin 500 mg qds Erythromycin 500 mg qds
Streptococcus pyogenes	Spreading infection, cellulitis, lymphangitis	Benzylpenicillin 600 mg bd Erythromycin 500 mg qds
Pseudomonas	Thick, foul-smelling green pus	Gentamicin 80 mg tds Ciprofloxacin 500 mg bd
Clostridium	Deep infection, necrosis, gangrene	Benzylpenicillin 600 mg bd Metronidazole 400 mg tds
Methicillin-resistant *Staph. aureus (MRSA)*	Slow-healing wounds	Vancomycin 500 mg qds IV Linezolid 60 mg bd

5. This lady had pes cavus as can be seen in Figure 40.3 that was confirmed by foot pressure measurement. She needed insoles to deflect pressure from her metatarsal heads. This was followed by the supply of a forefoot offloading sandal (Fig. 40.4). On return to clinic 6 weeks later, the lesion had healed (Fig. 40.5).

Key points

- Treatment of cellulitis demands immediate drainage of the septic lesion and appropriate antibiotic therapy, especially when spreading.
- The causative organism should be identified, as should the precise cause of the lesion.
- Pressure must be removed from areas of high load.

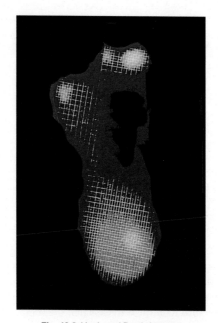

Fig. 40.3 Harris and Beath footprint

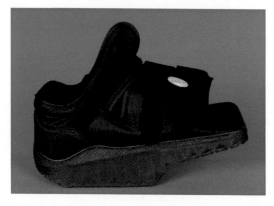

Fig. 40.4 Forefoot offloading sandal

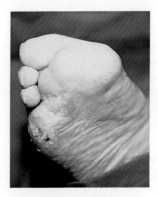

Fig. 40.5 Healed lesion

Further reading

Cunha BA (2000) Antibiotic selection for diabetic foot infections: a review. Journal of Foot and Ankle Surgery 39:253–7.

Van der Meer JWM, Koopmans PP, Lutterman JA (1996) Antibiotic therapy in diabetic foot infections. Diabetic Medicine August:48–51.

Case 41

The emergency medical services are called to the house of an 85-year-old lady who was found by a neighbour to be lying on the floor. She was subsequently diagnosed as having suffered a left hip fracture. Examination revealed that she had developed an ulcer on her heel (Fig. 41.1).

1. In what circumstances is ulceration of this type liable to develop?

2. What are the main treatment objectives?

3. How can adequate debridement of dead tissue be achieved?

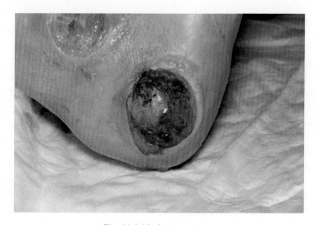

Fig. 41.1 Heel pressure sore

Pressure sores

1. Pressure ulcer development is most commonly found in patients who are medically 'compromised' with diminished skin perfusion. In effect, there has been a failure of the skin's normal barrier and temperature control functions, leading to a transcutaneous loss of fluid, electrolytes and protein. This process is exacerbated by changes associated with ageing, in particular the natural drying out of the skin secondary to diminished sebum production, and venous stasis. Although several pressure ulcer risk assessment tools are curently used by nurses, notably those of Waterlow, Braden and Gosnell, these are probably more beneficial in highlighting potential risk than in providing a true predictive value.

2. Normally the skin pH is acidic (4.0–5.5). Excessive use of substances that reduce its water-holding capacity, such as alkaline soaps, should be avoided and a well-balanced diet is necessary to optimize nutrition. Elevation will improve venous return and diminish swelling. It is extremely important to prevent further excoriation of the skin from abrasion and this will require padding around pressure points without causing any skin constriction. Air splints, sheepskin protectors and fluid mattresses will be helpful if available (Fig. 41.2).

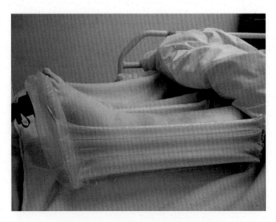

Fig. 41.2 Air splint to prevent heel pressure

3. Simple sores may be treated by regular wound dressing, applied as necessary. Necrotic tissue will need to be excised to leave a bleeding base. If direct excision is not feasible due to its extent, then larval therapy can be considered as shown in Figure 41.3.

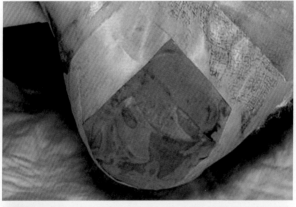

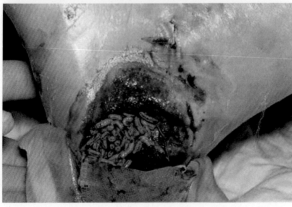

Fig. 41.3 Larval therapy

Key points

- Assess all patients for potential risk of pressure sores.
- Treat expeditiously, relieving pressure on the skin.
- Excise necrotic tissue.

Further reading

Benbow M (2007) Where is tissue viability in 2007? Journal of Community Nursing 21:34–8.

Jalali R, Rezaie M (2005) Predicting pressure ulcer risk: comparing the predictive validity of 4 scales. Advances in Skin and Wound Care 18:92–7.

Langemo D, Brown G (2006). Skin fails too: acute, chronic and end stage skin failure. Advances in Skin and Wound Care 19:206–12.

Section 6

Rheumatology

Case 42

A normal-looking woman complains that she repeatedly sprains her ankles. Examination reveals that she has marked pes planus and valgus hindfeet (Fig. 42.1). She has extremely flexible fingers, wrists, knees and spine (Fig. 42.2).

1. Diagnose this condition.
2. What heritable disorders of connective tissue should be excluded in your diagnosis?
3. How would you grade the severity of this young woman's condition?
4. What systemic sequelae are associated with this condition?
5. How should this condition be managed?
6. Specifically with regard to her feet, how should the problem of recurrent sprains be managed?

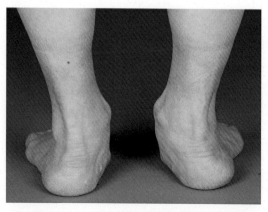

Fig. 42.1 Standing posterior view showing marked valgus alignment of both heels

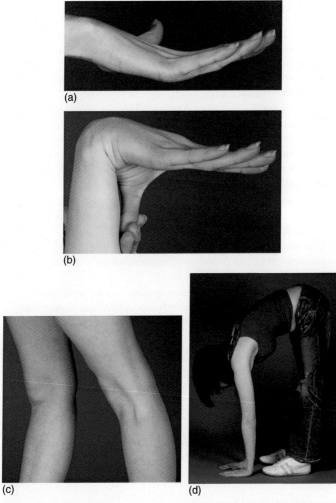

Fig. 42.2 (a) Hyperextension of metacarpal and proximal interphalangeal joints. (b) Wrist hyperflexion. (c) Hyperextension of knees. (d) Increased spinal flexibility

Benign joint hypermobility syndrome

1. Benign joint hypermobility syndrome (BJHS). Patients with BJHS show an increase in joint mobility. Sprains, subluxations and dislocations are common. Other musculoskeletal features include nerve compression disorders and early osteoarthritis.

2. Marfan's syndrome, Ehlers–Danlos syndrome and osteogenesis imperfecta are genetic diseases that include hypermobility as a feature. The skin hyperelasticity, hernias, lens anomalies and abnormal body proportions that typify these conditions are not present in patients with BJHS.

3. This patient scores 9/9 on the Beighton Scale (Table 42.1).

4. Mitral valve prolapse is more prevalent in patients with BJHS, as are uterine prolapse in women, varicose veins, bruising and generally poor wound healing.

5. Education on joint protection is important in BJHS. Strengthening and proprioceptive exercises are recommended to improve joint muscle function.

6. The tendency to recurrent ankle sprains may be lessened by use of antipronatory in-shoe orthoses. Additional supportive strapping or splinting may be helpful (Fig. 42.3).

Table 42.1 Criteria for joint hypermobility: the Beighton Scale (after Beighton et al 1983)

Item	Points
Passive dorsiflexion of little fingers beyond 90°	1 point each hand
Passive apposition of thumbs to flexor aspects of the forearms	1 point each hand
Hyperextension of knees beyond 10°	1 point each knee
Hyperextension of elbows beyond 10°	1 point each elbow
Forward flexion of the trunk, with knees straight, so the palms of hands rest easily on the floor	1 point

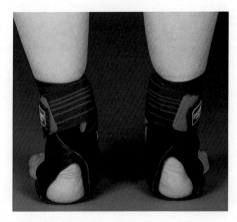

Fig. 42.3 Supportive strapping to improve ankle stability

Key points

- Patients with BJHS show an increase in joint mobility.
- Marfan's, Ehlers–Danlos and osteogenesis imperfecta are genetic diseases that include hypermobility as a feature.
- The Beighton Scale is used to grade the severity of this condition.
- Patients with BJHS may have additional health problems.
- Feet are often involved with BJHS and are treated with orthoses and supports.

Further reading

Adib N, Davies K, Grahame R, Woo P, Murray KJ (2005) Rheumatology joint hypermobility syndrome in childhood. A not so benign multisystem disorder. Rheumatology 44(6):744–50.

Beighton P, Grahame R, Bird H (1983) Assessment of hypermobility. In: Hypermobility of joints. Berlin: Springer-Verlag, 9–25.

Grahame R (2001) Time to take hypermobility seriously (in adults and children). Rheumatology 40:485–91.

Grahame R, Bird H (2001) British consultant rheumatologists' perceptions about hypermobility syndrome: a national survey. Rheumatology 40:559–62.

Russek LN (1999) Hypermobility syndrome. Physical Therapy 79:591–9.

Case 43

A young woman, in her early 20s, has persistent discomfort in the balls of both feet. Pain and stiffness are worse first thing in the morning. Her symptoms began insidiously, without a history of trauma. On examination, there is obvious swelling of the forefoot and the patient has become aware that her toes appear 'separated' (Fig. 43.1). Plantar skin lesions are shown in Figure 43.2.

1. This girl has an unusual presentation of metatarsalgia. Of what condition should you be suspicious and how frequently are feet affected with this condition?
2. What name is given to separation of the toes as seen in Figure 43.1?
3. Describe the diagnostic radiographic features in Figure 43.3. Is this a common site for this feature?
4. Name the further investigations which are now required.
5. What therapeutic measures should be considered?

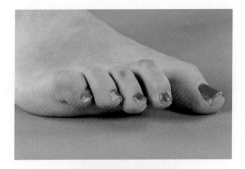

Fig. 43.1 Toe separation

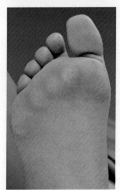

Fig. 43.2 Plantar skin lesions

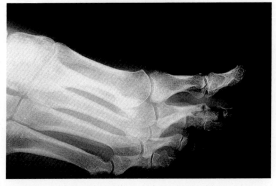

Fig. 43.3 Oblique radiograph of fifth MTP joint

Diagnosis of rheumatoid arthritis

1. In early presentation of rheumatoid arthritis, the feet are involved more frequently than the hands. Patients often complain of 'walking on pebbles'. Further examination will reveal swelling and tenderness in the MTP joints. These are painful when squeezed laterally.

2. Joint effusions can lead to spreading of toes, giving rise to the 'daylight sign'. Inflamed and full bursae are likely to be present over the metatarsal heads on the plantar side.

3. Radiographs of the feet show diagnostic erosions of the fifth metatarsal head. The metatarsal heads are the most common sites of erosive change, with an order of involvement from metatarsal 5, then 3, 2, 4 and 1. The metatarsal head erodes before the base of the proximal phalanx. The distal IP joints are rarely affected.

4. Investigations should include measurement of erythrocyte sedimentation rate (ESR), C-reactive protein (CRP), tests for rheumatoid factor and radiographs. Radiographs may be unremarkable in early disease (see also Table 43.1).

5. Disease-modifying antirheumatic drugs should be considered to retard the erosive process. Specific foot therapy is aimed at ensuring the patient's footwear is adequately wide at the toe box. Cushioning insoles will also help.

Key points

- Presentation of pain and swelling in the forefoot without a history of trauma should raise the suspicion of rheumatoid disease, particularly if accompanied by joint pain elsewhere.
- Feet are involved earlier and more frequently than the hands in rheumatoid arthritis.
- MTP joint erosions are diagnostic and indicate the need for second-line drug management.

Table 43.1 Laboratory findings in rheumatoid arthritis (based on Akil & Amos 1995)

Laboratory test	Abbreviation	Positive indication for RA	Normal values
Anaemia		(Normochromic or hypochromic, normocytic)	
Thrombocytosis			
• Serum iron concentration		Low	Male: <65 µg/dl Female: <50 µg/dl
• Low total iron binding capacity		Low	250–460 µg/dL
• Serum globulin		Raised	
• Serum alkaline phosphatase		Raised	
Acute phase response			
• Erythrocyte sedimentation rate	ESR	Raised	Male: 1–13 mm/h Female: 1–20 mm/h
• C-reactive protein concentration	CRP	Raised	<6 mg/l
Rheumatoid factor	RF	Present	Titres >1:80
Antinuclear antibodies	ANA	Present	Titres >1:80

Further reading

Akil M, Amos RS (1995) ABC of rheumatology: rheumatoid arthritis: clinical features. British Medical Journal 310:587–90.

Corbett M, Young A (1988) The Middlesex Hospital prospective study of early rheumatoid disease. British Rheumatology 27(suppl II):171–2.

Renton P (1991) Radiology of the foot. In: Disorders of the foot, 3rd edn. London: Blackwell Scientific Publications, 272–9.

Case 44

A 57-year-old woman is referred by her GP with a swelling on the dorsum of her left third toe. She has been aware of the swelling for some time but it is slowly getting bigger. The swelling was presumed to be a ganglion and so aspiration of the swelling was attempted. This was not successful although some blood-stained aspirate was noted. Her GP now thinks that she has a haemarthrosis, but would like a specialist opinion.

Examination of her left foot reveals a boggy, soft tissue mass on the dorsum of the left third toe (Fig. 44.1). The signs are not typical for a ganglion (see Fig. 10.1) and so an MR scan is requested (Fig. 44.2).

1. What are your differential diagnoses at this stage?
2. What features are revealed on MR imaging (see Fig. 44.2)?
3. How is the condition treated and what is the prognosis for this patient?

   How do the two conditions discussed in Question 1 differ?

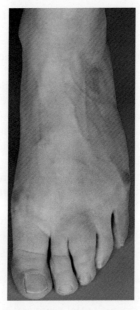

Fig. 44.1 Soft tissue swelling of the third toe

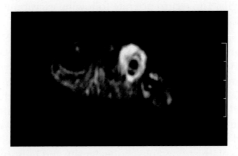

Fig. 44.2 MR scan of third toe: hyperintense mass centred on extensor tendon with extension onto plantar aspect of toe (T2-weighted image)

Pigmented villonodular synovitis/giant cell tumour of tendon sheath

1. The differential diagnoses were ganglion, chondroma, synovial chondromatosis, synovial sarcoma, pigmented villonodular synovitis (PVNS) and giant cell tumour of the tendon sheath (GCTTS). GCTTS was subsequently confirmed.

   GCTTS is an extra-articular process affecting tendon sheaths. It is an uncommon, locally aggressive disease characterized by the presence of hyperplastic synovium and presents as a painless, slowly growing soft tissue mass.

2. On MR imaging the hypervascularity and tendency to bleed result in the most characteristic finding of areas of signal void on all sequences due to paramagnetic effects of haemosiderin deposits. In this specific case, MR imaging shows a soft tissue mass on dorsal aspect of third toe. There is no bony involvement. The mass is centred around the extensor tendon but there is some extension onto the plantar aspect of the phalanx. The mass is hyper-intense on the water-weighted [T2] sequences and enhances diffusely.

3. Appropriate treatment is total synovectomy with histological confirmation of the diagnosis. Microscopic examination (Fig. 44.3) revealed synovial tissue in which there is a nodular and diffuse infiltrate of plump histiocytic cells with scattered lymphocytes and small numbers of osteoclast-like giant cells. The recurrence rate following excision may be up to 50%.

4. MR imaging and histological examination of GCTTS and PVNS are identical. GCTTS is extraarticular and PVNS is an intra-articular process that primarily affects single synovial joints, such as the knee, hip and ankle. As in GCTTS, in PVNS the onset is usually insidious, with patients complaining primarily of swelling but also stiffness around the affected joint. In contrast to GCTTS, PVNS will often show well-defined subchondral erosions and cysts with thin sclerotic rims on plain radiographs. Bone density and joint space are preserved.

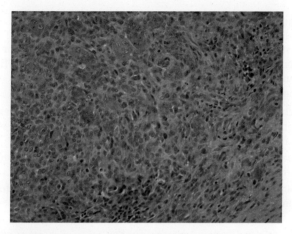

Fig. 44.3 Microscopy: histiocytic cells with scattered lymphocytes and small numbers of osteoclast-like giant cells

Key points

- GCTTS is an uncommon, locally aggressive disease characterized by hyperplastic synovium.
- MR images are important in diagnosing the condition as the sensitivity of MR detects haemosiderin deposition.
- Treatment is total synovectomy but recurrence rates following excision may be up to 50%.

Further reading

Carpintero P, Gascon E, Mesa M, Jimenez C, Lopez U (2007) Clinical and radiologic features of pigmented villonodular synovitis of the foot: report of eight cases. Journal of the American Podiatric Medicine Association 97(5):415–19.

Foo LF, Raby N (2005) Tumours and tumour-like lesions of the foot and ankle. Clinical Radiology 60(3):308–32.

Frassica FJ, Bhimani MA, McCarthy EF, Wenz J (1999) Pigmented villonodular synovitis of the hip and knee. American Family Physician 60(5):1404–15.

Ganley TJ, De Ruiter CJ, Dormans JP, Meyer JS, Collins MH (1998) Ankle pain and swelling in a 10-year-old girl. Clinical Orthopaedics and Related Research 348:282–9.

Case 45

After stepping off a pavement awkwardly, a middle-aged doctor suddenly found that her great toe became extremely painful. There was little to observe initially, but during the next week severe swelling developed (Fig. 45.1).

1. Why was the doctor's toe swollen and inflamed? What other conditions may mimic this inflammatory arthropathy and what is its most likely cause?

2. How can the condition be diagnosed in the laboratory? Would a negative blood test exclude the condition?

3. Various treatments are recommended, but which is best? How long should therapy continue?

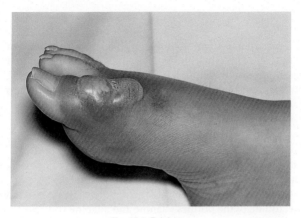

Fig. 45.1 Painful toe

Gout

1. The description is typical of that of a patient with tophaceous gout (Fig. 45.2). The condition generally affects men in middle age, but is not uncommon in women after the menopause. Prevalence is higher in some racial groups such as the Maori and African Americans.

   Chondrocalcinosis, or pseudogout, rarely affects the foot and ankle as calcium pyrophosphate dihydrate crystals are preferentially laid down in articular fibrocartilage or the cartilage at the sites of ligamentous attachments to bone (in the knee, wrist, pubic symphysis and intervertebral discs).

   Gout is caused by an elevated serum urate. This is a natural metabolite of the purines guanine and adenine (nucleic acid components), and hence any condition increasing the rate of purine breakdown, or restricting urate excretion, may precipitate gout. For lack of a more obvious cause, the condition is often attributed to a dietary excess, including high alcohol and/or seafood consumption. It is worthwhile

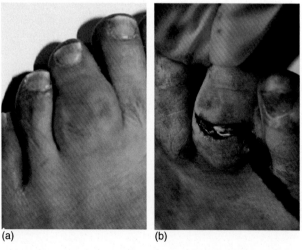

(a)   (b)

Fig. 45.2 Gouty tophus infiltrating third toe and exuding urate on incision

screening patients at their initial attack for any blood disorder causing excessive nucleoprotein production. The practitioner should also ensure that the patient is not on a diuretic altering renal urate filtration.

2. Monosodium urate monohydrate precipitates out to form either an amorphous mass or needle-shaped crystals of 0.2–2 µm in length (Fig. 45.3). A definitive diagnosis will be reached if crystals can be visualized and generally the affected joint must be aspirated. Serum urate levels will not always reflect the severity of the condition. The chance of a patient suffering gout does increase if the urate is elevated above normal (>420 µmol/l in males or 380 µmol/l in females), but many patients will maintain normal urate levels outwith their acute attacks.

3. Non-steroidal anti-inflammatory drugs which inhibit cyclo-oxygenase (the enzyme that converts arachidonic acid to prostaglandins) provide analgesia and an anti-inflammatory effect in acute gout. Salicylate (aspirin) is contraindicated, but colchicine may be considered (0.5 mg 2 hourly until the acute attack settles). An intra-articular corticosteroid injection will sometimes provide temporary symptomatic relief if only one joint is inflamed.

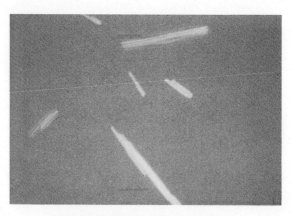

Fig. 45.3 Negatively birefringent urate crystals

For long-term prevention of recurrent attacks, either uricosuric agents such as probenecid and sulphinpyrazone or the xanthine oxidase inhibitor allopurinol are required. Maintenance doses of allopurinol (200–600 mg daily) are required for life.

Key points

- Acute gout may be precipitated by trauma or low temperature as these will facilitate crystallization. Peripheral joints are frequently affected.
- Monosodium urate needles are negatively birefringent when viewed under polarized light.
- Allopurinol should not be used as primary treatment for acute gout.

Further reading

Davis JC (1999) A practical approach to gout. Current management of an 'old' disease. Postgraduate Medicine 106:115-16, 119–23.

Sturrock R (2000) Gout. Easy to misdiagnose. British Medical Journal 320:132–3.

Case 46

Foot problems are only one element of the condition affecting this 25-year-old man. As well as a recent history of plantar and posterior heel pain (Fig. 46.1), he also has a history of non-specific urethritis.

1. This condition usually presents as a triad of symptoms. What are they?
2. Who does this syndrome affect, and what is the usual precursor?
3. Enthesitis is a feature of this syndrome. What is it and where does it occur?
4. Arthritis affects mainly which joints and how are they treated?
5. What is the skin lesion shown in Figure 46.2?

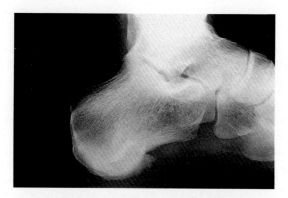

Fig. 46.1 Lateral radiograph of the hindfoot

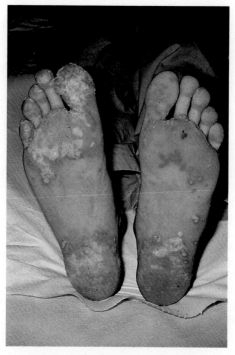

Fig. 46.2 Skin lesions on the sole of the foot

Reiter's syndrome

1. Reiter's syndrome comprises a triad of symptoms: seronegative arthritis, conjunctivitis and non-specific urethritis. Although originally described as this triad, Reiter's disease can still reasonably be diagnosed if one component, usually conjunctivitis, is absent. Other symptoms may also be present, notably balanitis, stomatitis and keratoderma. Some of these give only mild and temporary discomfort.

2. Reiter's syndrome is found in men 13 times more frequently than in women, the age of onset being between 20 and 30 years. The usual precursor is a urogenital or enteric infection, particularly with *Chlamydia trachomatis*. As with the other seronegative arthropathies, there is an association with the HLA-B27 antigen.

3. Enthesopathy, which is an inflammation at the attachment of fascia, ligaments and tendons to bone (entheses) such as the Achilles tendon and plantar fascia, occurs early but is persistent. Sacroiliitis and spondylitis will develop in susceptible individuals. Initially, only soft tissue swelling may be observed radiologically but eventually erosions will be visible and finally, reactive bone sclerosis. This is characterized in patients with plantar heel pain by the formation of calcaneal spurs that are large and have ill-defined margins. They are described as 'fluffy' in appearance. Erosions also occur at the posterior surface of the calcaneus at the attachment of the Achilles tendon.

4. One joint at a time becomes swollen, with the lower limbs affected more often than the upper. The predilection is for the knees, ankles and toes. The pattern of joint disease is that of a transient, asymmetrical polyarthritis, which develops acutely, subsiding after a few weeks. However, some cases progress to a more chronic relapsing and remitting form of disabling arthritis. Aspiration of swollen joints may be required and corticosteroid injection may be helpful. Non-steroidal anti-inflammatory drugs are generally prescribed, but some patients require sulphasalazine or other disease-modifying antirheumatic drugs.

5. Involvement of the skin of the soles of the feet is termed keratoderma blennorrhagicum. The lesions appear first as brown macules but they rapidly develop into painless, reddened, often confluent raised plaques and pustules. They are similar, both clinically and histologically to the lesions of pustular psoriasis. Toenails become dystrophic which can cause them to separate off, with regrowth after 3–6 months. Keratoderma is helped by the application of hydrocortisone cream.

Key points

- Reiter's syndrome is a triad of seronegative arthritis, conjunctivitis and non-specific urethritis.
- Enthesopathy is a common feature and can affect the plantar fascia and insertion of the Achilles tendon.
- Keratoderma blennorrhagicum affects the soles of the feet.

Further reading

Conska GW (1987) Reiter's syndrome. Update 15 December:1284–94.

Tozzi MA, Stamm R, Bigelli A, Hart D (1981) Reiter's syndrome: a review and case report. Journal of the American Podiatric Medicine Association 71:418–22.

Yi-Kettula UI (1984) Clinical characteristics in male and female Reiter's syndrome. Clinical Rheumatology 3:351–60.

Case 47

The nails hold the key to the diagnosis of this man's painful foot. He is 32 years old and was presumed to have a fungal infection of his right great toenail despite negative mycology. He now presents in clinic with an acutely painful and swollen right great toe (Fig. 47.1). He also complains of pain in his right heel and ring finger of his right hand. On close examination there is pitting of his fingernails (Fig. 47.2).

1. Explain why mycology was normal in this case.
2. Which radiological features are evident on inspection of the radiograph in Figure 47.3?
3. Given the clinical and radiological presentation, which condition is this?
4. Which digit is most commonly affected and which other joints may be involved?
5. What might a radiograph of the heel reveal?

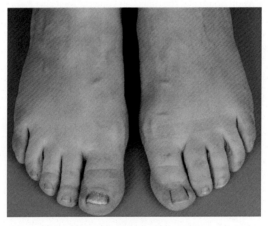

Fig. 47.1 Swollen right great toe with thickened toenail

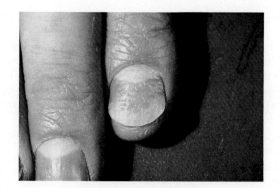

Fig. 47.2 Pitting of the finger nails

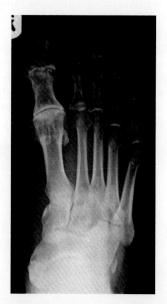

Fig. 47.3 Radiograph: periarticular erosions of the first IP joint

Psoriatic arthritis

1. The nail disease in this case is due to psoriasis, not fungal infection (see Fig. 27.1). The patient may have skin lesions over the extensor aspects of the elbows and knees, but skin involvement may be minimal or hidden, such as pitting of the nails or flaking of the scalp. Separation of the nail from the nail bed (onycholysis) is another typical feature of psoriasis.

2. The radiograph in Figure 47.3 reveals periarticular erosions at the first IP joint.

3. Psoriatic arthritis is a seronegative joint disease mainly affecting the small peripheral joints and the spine (spondyloarthropathy). The pattern of joint disease illustrated in this case is described as an asymmetrical oligoarthritis involving scattered small joints, giving rise to 'sausage' digits (dactylitis) (see Fig. 47.1). Psoriatic arthritis may also present as a type that is indistinguishable from rheumatoid arthritis, or as the rare but very destructive arthritis mutilans (Fig. 47.4).

4. Psoriatic arthritis most commonly affects the great toe, but radiological changes may be seen at any of the IP joints. There is a tendency for the condition to involve the feet before the hands. More severe disease brings about 'pencil and cup' deformities. Joint ankylosis may occur secondary to a periostitis

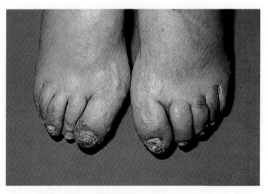

Fig. 47.4 Arthritis mutilans of the foot

that causes new bone to be laid down along the joint margins. This is the primary cause of sacroiliitis.

5. Inflammation at the origin of the plantar fascia commonly presents as a painful heel. Radiographs often reveal large heel spurs that have irregular and ill-defined cortical margins (see Fig. 46.1). The enthesopathy can be accompanied by insertional Achilles tendinopathy (see Fig. 62.1).

Key points

- Psoriatic arthritis affects the joints of the hands, feet and spine.
- Skin involvement may be hidden.
- Psoriatic arthritis can present as a very destructive arthritis mutilans.
- Heel spurs are large with an irregular cortical outline.

Further reading

Gerster JC, Piccinin P (1984) Enthesopathy of the heels in juvenile onset seronegative B-27 positive spondyloarthropathy. Journal of Rheumatology 12:310–14.

Kingsley G, Pugh N (2004) Spondyloarthropathies. In: ABC of rheumatology, 3rd edn. London: BMJ Publishing, 61–7.

Renton P (1991) Radiology of the foot. In: Disorders of the foot, 3rd edn. London: Blackwell Scientific Publications, 272–9.

Case 48

The foot is involved in most patients with rheumatoid arthritis. An elderly lady with established rheumatoid disease repeatedly attends the podiatry clinic (Fig. 48.1).

1. Describe the pathological changes that have taken place to result in this forefoot deformity.
2. How is the rest of the foot affected with rheumatoid arthritis?
3. How should this patient be managed?
4. Is there a role for surgery here?
5. Which non-articular features of rheumatoid arthritis are sometimes found in the foot and lower limb?

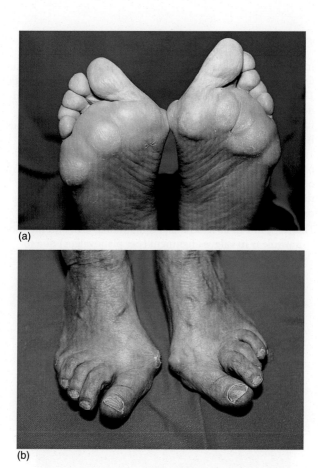

(a)

(b)

Fig. 48.1 (a, b) Plantar and dorsal aspects of rheumatoid foot

Therapy of rheumatoid arthritis

1. In established rheumatoid disease, there are a number of classic features. These include hallux valgus (90%) and joint subluxation. The joints often become subluxed and the toes become clawed due to fixed flexion deformities of the joints. The plantar-fibrofatty pad, which is intended to protect the metatarsal heads, is pulled distally and exposes the metatarsal heads (Fig. 48.2). The prominence of the metatarsal heads in turn leads to high pressures, resultant bursae and plantar callosities. A combination of increased local pressure and relative ischaemia creates a risk of ulceration and secondary infection. Figure 48.3 shows osteoporosis, bone destruction and deformity.

2. There is a low or absent medial longitudinal arch and the foot as a whole is in valgus alignment (pes planovalgus) due to

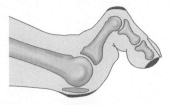

Fig. 48.2 Prolapse of the metatarsal heads in rheumatoidal arthritis

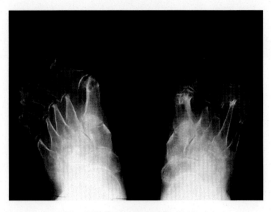

Fig. 48.3 Radiograph of the forefoot

collapse of the subtalar joint. Synovitis, articular erosion and stretching of the ligaments has allowed the talar head to adduct and plantarflex with resultant bulging of the foot medially. This posture of the foot in rheumatoid arthritis is often exacerbated by valgus alignment of the knee and there may be impingement between the talus and fibula. Excessive pronation of the foot also places a strain on tibialis posterior (stance phase inverter of the foot) which may rupture. Gait tends to be antalgic and apropulsive, with a prolonged double support stance phase. The ankle joint is less frequently involved in rheumatoid arthritis.

3. Soft insoles relieve pressure from the painful metatarsal heads (Fig. 48.4). Orthoses are valuable to improve the alignment of the foot and to relieve forefoot pressure (see evidence box below). Bespoke or semi-bespoke footwear is important to accommodate hallux valgus and digital deformities. These can be modified with a Thomas heel and medial heel flare to create medial stability, which has been lost with progressive valgus alignment of the foot.

4. Surgical management is aimed at relieving forefoot pressure, usually by some form of excisional or replacement arthroplasty of the forefoot. Additional operations for the rheumatoid foot include triple arthrodesis of the hindfoot to produce a more plantigrade foot, arthrodesis of the ankle, tibialis posterior repair and selective toe surgery.

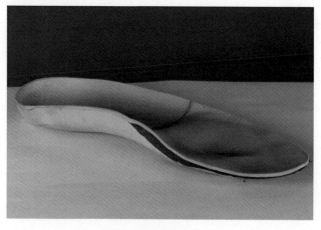

Fig. 48.4 Soft insole

5. Vasculitis occurs in patients with high titres of rheumatoid factor and severe erosive disease. Vasculitic ulcers tend to be deep with sharp margins ('punched out'). They occur anywhere on the leg and foot, but are more common on the lower leg (Fig. 48.5). These ulcers are painful and difficult to treat. They generally occur during the active stages of the disease and require disease-modifying antirheumatic drugs.

    Subcutaneous nodules are present in 20% of patients with rheumatoid arthritis. These feel firm, non-tender and are freely movable, although they can be attached to deeper structures. In the foot they occur over the MTP joints, around the Achilles tendon and on the extensor surface of the toes.

Evidence

One RCT has demonstrated that custom-designed foot orthoses used continuously over a 30-month treatment period resulted in a reduction of foot pain by 19.1%, foot disability by 30.8%, and functional limitation by 13.5%. The authors also concluded that clinical effectiveness might be enhanced by their use in the early stages of rearfoot pain and deformity.

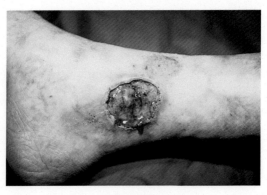

Fig. 48.5 Vasculitic ulceration

Key points

- The forefoot is the source of great discomfort to patients with rheumatoid arthritis.
- The metatarsal heads become prominent and are subjected to excessive pressure which increases the risk of ulceration.
- Palliative insoles and suitable footwear are essential.
- Vasculitis and nodules occur in aggressive disease.

Further reading

Klenerman L (1995) The foot and ankle in rheumatoid arthritis. Rheumatology 34:443–8.

Thomas S, Kinninmonth AWG, Kumar SC (2006) Long-term results of the modified Hoffman procedure in the rheumatoid forefoot: surgical technique. Journal of Bone and Joint Surgery 88 A(suppl 1):149–57.

Woodburn J, Barker S, Helliwell PS (2002) A randomized controlled trial of foot orthoses in rheumatoid arthritis. Journal of Rheumatology 29(7):1377–83.

Woodburn J, Helliwell PS, Barker S (2002) Three-dimensional kinematics at the ankle joint complex in rheumatoid arthritis patients with painful valgus deformity of the rearfoot. Rheumatology 41:1406–12.

Section 7

Neurology

Case 49

This patient regularly has to remove her shoe while shopping. She is a 45-year-old research worker who presents with a sharp, shooting pain in the ball of her left foot and toes. The pain began as a burning, tingling sensation, which is now more intense and neuralgic in nature. She is only able to walk short distances. Relief of pain can be aided by massaging her foot or manipulating her toes. On examination, there is a sensory deficit in the region demonstrated in Figure 49.1. Pain is exacerbated by lateral compression of her forefoot (Fig. 49.2).

1. Name this condition and state the group of patients most commonly affected by it.
2. Which test is being carried out in Figure 49.2 and precisely where would you expect to localize pain?
3. Name additional investigations that are helpful in confirming a diagnosis.
4. Discuss the aetiology of this condition.
5. Outline a treatment plan for this patient.

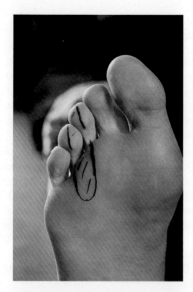

Fig. 49.1 Area of sensory deficit affecting the toes

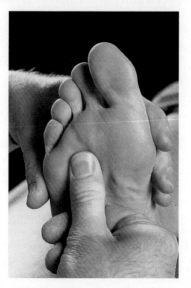

Fig. 49.2 Clinical examination of the foot

Morton's neuroma

1. Morton's neuroma is a common, paroxysmal neuralgia affecting the web spaces of the toes. Pain arises from a pathological plantar digital nerve as it divides to supply the adjacent sides of the toes it innervates. Presentation can be bilateral and often there are two lesions in the same foot. Middle-aged women are most commonly affected.

2. Using a thumb, firm pressure applied to the affected web space will elicit focal tenderness which may be exacerbated by simultaneously compressing the metatarsal heads together (see Fig. 49.2). This may be accompanied by a painful 'Mulder's click'. The third web space is most frequently involved, followed by the second. Symptoms never occur in either the first or fourth web spaces. The exact site of tenderness is located to a point between and just anterior to the heads of the two adjacent metatarsals. Other clinical signs and symptoms are summarized in Table 49.1.

3. Ultrasonography is routinely used to detect neuroma. A typical sonographic appearance is that of a hypoechoic mass (varying in density from the surrounding tissue), orientated parallel to the long axis of the metatarsals (Fig. 49.3). Although the validity of ultrasound scans has been questioned, our approach is to confirm a swelling on the nerve with ultrasound before operation.

Table 49.1 Summary of the clinical signs and symptoms of Morton's neuroma

Subjective symptoms	Objective symptoms
• Sharp, lancing or cramp-like pain often likened to a burning hot needle	• Pain located in second or third web space elicited with plantar pressure and exacerbated by lateral compression
• Pain only on walking	• Painful Mulder's click present
• Patient has to stop walking	• Loss of sharp sensation between toes
• Patient has to rest until pain goes (relief aided by removing shoes and massaging toes)	• Injection of local anaesthetic temporarily ameliorates pain
• Pins and needles or numbness experienced between toes	

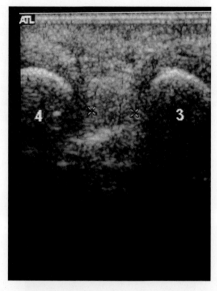

Fig. 49.3 Ultrasound scan of the intermetatarsal spaces showing a swelling on the plantar digital nerve to the third and fourth toes

4. Histological changes are consistent with an entrapment neuropathy of the plantar digital nerve. Constrictive footwear is implicated as the main causative factor in compressing the nerve. This is substantiated by the relief of pain found on shoe removal and the higher occurrence of the condition in women. Young people rarely develop a Morton's neuroma suggesting that degenerative fibrosis may be one contributing factor.

5. Conservative management starts with advice to the patient to change the style of their shoes. Broad, lace-up shoes are to be recommended and high-heeled, slip-on court shoes avoided. Insoles can only be considered if the footwear will accommodate them, or they will worsen the problem. Insoles such as metatarsal dome support will lift and spread the metatarsals. Orthoses can be used to reduce forefoot hypermobility.

An injection of corticosteroid is the third line of treatment. The evidence shows that this is effective but a recurrence of symptoms should be expected. If patients have a good response to an initial injection, then a second or even a third injection is possible but the risk of subcutaneous fat atrophy and hypopigmentation increases (see Fig. 49.4). There is only limited evidence for the use of alcohol injections. Beyond this, surgery has to be considered (Fig. 49.5). A dorsal incision is probably preferable as it avoids the risk of a troublesome scar and also allows early postoperative weightbearing.

A four-stage treatment plan is summarized in Figure 49.6.

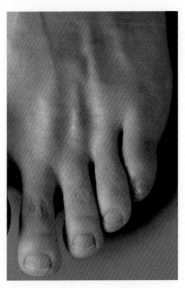

Fig. 49.4 Atrophy of subcutaneous tissue following steroid injection

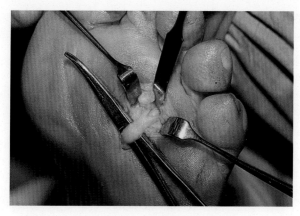

Fig. 49.5 Excision of the plantar digital nerve through a plantar incision

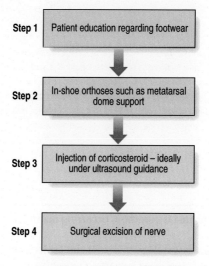

Step 1	Patient education regarding footwear
Step 2	In-shoe orthoses such as metatarsal dome support
Step 3	Injection of corticosteroid – ideally under ultrasound guidance
Step 4	Surgical excision of nerve

Fig. 49.6 Four-stage treatment plan

Clinical tip: corticosteroid injection for Morton's neuroma

Injection of corticosteroid is a standard treatment for Morton's neuroma.

Solution/volume	Methyl prednisolone 0.5 ml (20 mg) and lignocaine hydrochloride 1 ml (2%)
Needle	A 25 gauge (blue) or 27 gauge (long) needle is ideal
Technique of injection	Locate the painful intermetatarsal space, invariably the second or third. Identify the metatarsal heads and, from the dorsum, introduce the needle just proximal to the level of the metatarsal heads. Penetrate until resistance of the plantar skin is met. Withdraw the needle about 0.5 cm, aspirating to avoid intravascular injection, and then inject half the volume of contents of the syringe. Withdraw the needle a further 0.5 cm and inject the remainder

Evidence

A systematic Cochrane review concluded that there is insufficient evidence with which to assess the effectiveness of surgical and non-surgical interventions for Morton's neuroma. Subsequently one randomized controlled trial of 125 patients has demonstrated that a single injection under ultrasound guidance is effective in the treatment of this condition at 3 months, but that this is not of long-standing benefit. Concurrently an economic analysis showed that this treatment may not be cost effective. The literature suggests a success rate of 70–80% for surgical excision of the nerve.

Key points

- Morton's neuroma is common, occurring mainly in the third web space.
- Pain is characteristically paroxysmal and limits walking.
- Footwear is the dominant causative factor.
- Management is directed at advice on footwear, use of insoles and corticosteroid injections.
- Excision of the nerve remains the mainstay of treatment.

Further reading

Fanucci E, Masala S, Fabiano S et al (2004) Treatment of intermetatarsal Morton's neuroma with alcohol injection under US guide: 10 month follow-up. European Radiology 14(3):514–18.

Hassouna H, Dingh D, Taylor H, Johnson S (2007) Ultrasound guided steroid injection in the treatment of interdigital neuralgia. Acta Orthopaedica Belgica 73(2):224–9.

Hughes RJ, Ali K, Jones H, Kendall S, Connell DA (2007) Treatment of Morton's neuroma with alcohol injection under sonographic guidance: follow-up of 101 cases. Am J Roentgenol 188(6):1535–9.

Sharp RJ, Wade CM, Hennessy MS, Saxby TS (2003) The role of MRI and ultrasound imaging in Morton's neuroma and the effect of size of lesion on symptoms. Journal of Bone and Joint Surgery 85(7):999–1005.

Thomson CE, Martin D, Gibson JNA (2004) Treatment interventions for Morton's neuroma: a systematic review. Cochrane Database of Systematic Reviews, Issue 3.

Thomson CE, Beggs I, Martin D et al (2007) Focus on Research. Steroid injections (methylprednisolone) in the treatment of Morton's neuroma: patient-blind randomised trial. Scottish Executive Health Department, Chief Scientist's Office. Available online at www.sehd.scot.nhs.uk:80/cso/index.htm.

Case 50

This single 25-year-old man would like to wear a kilt! Unfortunately he is extremely self conscious about the appearance of his leg (Fig. 50.1), supposedly injured as a young child when he fell off the back of a motorcycle whilst growing up in India. There was no evidence of any proximal injury. On further questioning, he is aware that as a child he had been quite ill with a fever. Functionally, he has a 5 cm limb length discrepancy although he walks reasonably well despite a flail right foot. He has been helped with surgery in childhood (Fig. 50.2) but he has a residual calcaneus deformity. On the right side he weight bears only on his heel (note the hypertrophy of the heel pad; Fig. 50.3). He is now living in the UK and seeks help with the cosmetic appearance of his right leg.

1. Why is the account of his leg injury unlikely and what is a more feasible explanation for the deformity apparent in Figures 50.1–3?
2. Which clinical investigations are required to confirm this diagnosis?
3. Which operations have been performed on his right foot?
4. What conservative measures could be offered to help this young man?

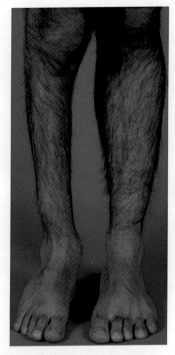

Fig. 50.1 Limb asymmetry

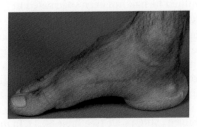

Fig. 50.2 Medial scar and hypertrophic heel

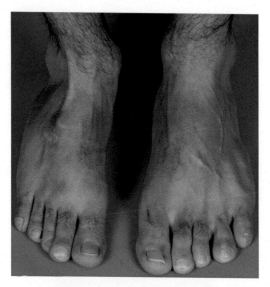

Fig. 50.3 Re-routed tibialis posterior tendon

Poliomyelitis

1. His story does not add up, as an injury to his right ankle would not account for the absence of calf muscle bulk or the degree of shortness of the right leg. A more plausible explanation, given the presenting features and the fact that he had a febrile episode, is that he had contracted poliomyelitis. Later his parents admitted he had not been vaccinated in India.

2. Neurological investigations are required to examine the man's posture, muscle bulk, tone and power, plus his co-ordination and reflexes. The most striking feature is the lack of symmetry, due to lack of calf muscle bulk on his right side. Hypotonia (flaccidity) or decreased tone is readily apparent. Power or strength may be tested by comparing a patient's strength against your own, comparing one side to the other and grading strength using the Medical Research Council (MRC) scale (see Table 50.1). In this case the anterior group of muscles were weak with an MRC score of 0 and reflexes were absent, indicating a lower motor neuron lesion.

Table 50.1 MRC scale

Grade	Description
0	No contraction
1	Flicker or trace of contraction
2	Active movement with gravity eliminated
3	Active movement against gravity
4	Active movement against gravity and resistance
5	Normal power

3. Because of anterior muscle weakness, an attempt has been made to use the tibialis posterior as a dorsiflexor by transferring it through the intraosseous membrane onto the dorsum of the foot. His right heel has gone into valgus as a consequence of losing normal tibialis posterior action.

4. The simplest approach would be to supply a heel raise by use of an insole and heel lift to address the limb length discrepancy. A prosthesis could also be offered to go inside his kilt sock to improve cosmesis. This patient was not content with these simple measures and wanted to be considered for leg lengthening and silicone implant insertion within his calf.

Key points

- Consider previous polio as a cause of muscle weakness and calf atrophy.
- Muscle strength can be graded on the MRC scale.
- Tendon transfers aim to restore muscle balance and improve gait.

Clinical tip:

1. A transferred muscle loses at least one grade in power.
2. The muscle transferred must be strong enough to replace the paralysed muscle.
3. Agonists work better than antagonists.
4. Transferred tendons should pass through a sheath to allow glide.
5. Innervation and blood supply must be retained.
6. Tendons will only move 'normal' joints.
7. Transferred tendons must have adequate tension.
8. A similar range of excursion is desirable.

Further reading

Mestikawy M, Zeier F (1971) Tendon transfers for poliomyelitis. Clinical Orthopaedics and Related Research 75:188–94.

Perry J, Barnes G, Gronley JK (1988) The postpolio syndrome: an overuse phenomenon. Clinical Orthopaedics and Related Research 233:145–62.

Song HR, Myrboh V, Oh CW, Lee ST, Lee SH (2005) Tibial lengthening and concomitant foot deformity correction in 14 patients with permanent deformity after poliomyelitis. Acta Orthopaedica Scandinavica 76(2):261–9.

Turner JW, Cooper R (1972) Anterior transfer of the tibialis posterior through the interosseus membrane. Clinical Orthopaedics and Related Research 83:241–4.

Case 51

A 45-year-old man has type I insulin-dependent diabetes mellitus. He presents with a painless plantar ulcer (Fig. 51.1).

1. What are the main factors that lead to foot ulceration in diabetes mellitus?
2. What investigations are appropriate?
3. How would you manage this patient?

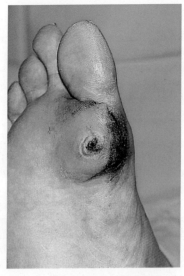

Fig. 51.1 Plantar ulceration

Diabetic neuropathic ulcer

1. The principal factor that leads to foot ulcers in patients with diabetes is neuropathy. Excessive plantar pressure and trauma are also significant causative factors, with atherosclerosis as a contributory factor.

2. The priority for assessment of this patient is to establish which of the following prevails.

a) *Neuropathy*

Motor neuropathy. Gross inspection of the foot may reveal an abnormal arch and clawing of the toes, indicating intrinsic muscle wastage. Structural changes affect foot function and altered loading, and this is reflected in the presence of plantar callouses.

Sensory neuropathy. In the presence of plantar ulceration there will be decreased perception of pain across the forefoot and this patient demonstrated a loss of sharp/blunt discrimination. Semi-quantitative assessment of light touch can be obtained using a 10 g Semmes-Weinstein monofilament. Loss of vibration can be performed using a 128 Hz tuning fork. To give a quantitative assessment, a neurothesiometer may be used.

Patients with diabetes mellitus typically present with sensory loss in a 'glove and stocking' distribution. Joint proprioception is absent and consequently the body does not adapt to excessive stresses placed across the foot and ankle joints. Articular cartilage destruction and bone erosion swiftly follow, leading to destroyed insensate Charcot joints (Fig. 51.2). It is important, therefore, to X-ray the entire foot and ankle. Radiological features will include both destructive and hypertrophic changes. Often, there will be marked loss of the affected joint spaces, with fragmentation and resorption of subchondral bone and osteophyte formation.

Autonomic neuropathy. This is apparent if the skin is dry and flaky, and perhaps also by distension of the dorsal veins, which is a sign of arteriovenous shunting which can lead to changes in blood flow and result in a net loss of bone contributing to joint neuropathy.

b) *Arteriopathy*

Gangrene is indicative of ischaemia and is illustrated in Figure 51.3. Thrombosis of the digital arteries has led to gangrene of the toe. It is often secondary to infection,

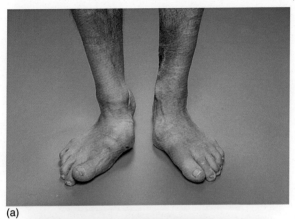

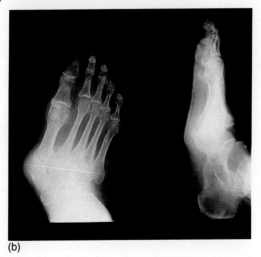

Fig. 51.2 (a) Clinical appearance and (b) radiograph of Charcot joints.

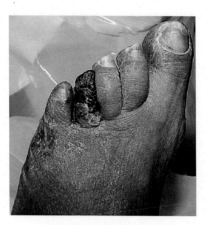

Fig. 51.3 Digital gangrene

which in this case involves both the soft tissues and phalanx. If the lesion is dry then the digit can be left to autoamputate but this lesion was malodorous and required amputation and antibiotic therapy.

Assessment of arterial disease predicts the outcome of ulcer healing. If the foot is found to be sufficiently ischaemic then the ulcer will not heal. Ankle brachial pressure indices (Fig. 37.2) are important in assessment but the clinician should be mindful of the caveat of a raised index due to Mönckeberg's sclerosis (arteriolar calcification) when, due to arteriovenous shunting, blood short-circuits the toes. The latter is detectable with a hand-held Doppler ultrasound probe as a loud, monotone signal. Digital systolic pressures can be measured with a toe cuff (Fig. 51.4). A normal toe:brachial index is >0.7.

c) *Infection*

Cellulitis will be accompanied by inflammation, although if the blood supply is compromised then this may not be obvious. Deep probing of the wound is required to exclude deep infection that will require surgical drainage and excision of any necrotic tissue. Bone destruction, sequestrum formation and subperiosteal new bone are radiological features of osteomyelitis.

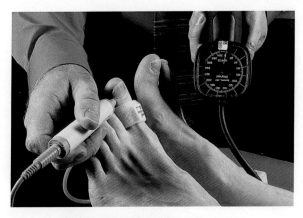

Fig. 51.4 Digital systolic pressure measurement

3. The clinician should have two aims. Firstly, it is essential
to prevent spread of infection from the ulcer and it should
be immediately debrided of all necrotic tissue and a broad-
spectrum antibiotic prescribed. Later, to encourage vascularity,
the wound may be dressed with a hydrogel, hydrocolloid
or alginate as appropriate. Secondly, to prevent recurrent
ulcer formation, and indeed generally before healing can be
established at all, the plantar pressure must be redistributed.
In this case an Aircast® walker (Fig. 51.5) was used, but a total-
contact plaster shoe would probably have worked just as well.
In the longer term, diabetic insoles and footwear (Fig. 51.6),
together with regular visits to a podiatrist, are essential.

Evidence

A systematic review has revealed some evidence, from one large trial, that a
screening and foot protection programme reduces the rate of major amputations.
The evidence for special footwear and educational programmes is equivocal.
There is evidence from one trial that podiatric care significantly reduces callous
formation.

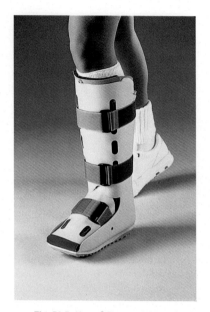

Fig. 51.5 Aircast® Pneumatic Walker

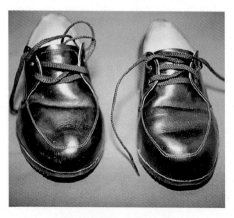

Fig. 51.6 Bespoke footwear

Key points

- Neuropathic joints lead to gross deformity in the diabetic foot.
- The insensate diabetic foot is at risk of ulceration from increased plantar pressures. This, combined with peripheral vascular disease, leads to poor wound healing and increases the risk of infection.
- Assessment of diabetic ulceration must include assessment of infection, neuropathy and arteriopathy.
- Healing of neuropathic ulcers is established by relief of high pressures and careful wound care.

Further reading

Edmonds M, Blundell M, Morris H (1986) The diabetic foot: impact of a foot clinic. Quarterly Journal of Medicine 232:763–71.

Edwards J (2002) Debridement of diabetic foot ulcers. Cochrane Database of Systematic Reviews, Issue 4.

O'Meara S, Cullum N, Majid M, Sheldon T (2000) Systematic reviews of wound care management: (3) antimicrobial agents for chronic wounds; (4) diabetic foot ulceration. Health Technology Assessment 4(21).

Singh N, Armstrong DG, Lipsky B (2005) Preventing foot ulcers in patients with diabetes. Journal of the American Medical Association 293(2):217–28.

Spencer S (2001) Pressure relieving interventions for preventing and treating diabetic foot ulcers (Cochrane Review). In: The Cochrane Library Issue 2. Oxford: Update Software.

Case 52

A young boy presents to the clinic after his mother noted that his right foot had a higher arch than his left (Fig. 52.1). She stated that he had never played sport, as he was rather 'clumsy' and unco-ordinated with poor balance. Examination revealed that his calves were thin, especially in comparison with his thighs where his muscles were clearly well developed. In addition, he had slight weakness of intrinsic muscle power in both hands.

1. Why should this boy's father be examined?
2. What tests are valuable in establishing his diagnosis?
3. If he had presented at 40 years of age, would his diagnosis have been different?
4. Will any form of therapy be beneficial and what other deformities may develop?
5. Will the boy have a normal life expectancy?

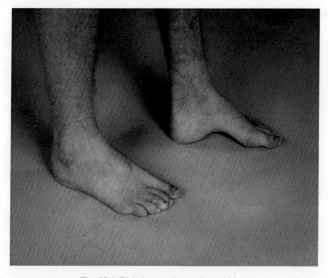

Fig. 52.1 Right leg wasting and cavoid foot

Hereditary motor and sensory neuropathy (HMSN)

1. The patient presents with a progressive wasting disorder causing weakness of the peroneal muscles and a cavoid foot. At this age of onset the condition is probably type I HMSN (classically referred to as peroneal muscular atrophy or Charcot–Marie–Tooth disease), although several other similar conditions have been described. Charcot–Marie–Tooth is an autosomal dominant condition and therefore a familial trait would be expected.

2. Generally, the peripheral nerves are palpable and, on electrophysiological testing, there will be marked slowing of motor and sensory nerve conduction velocities. Muscle biopsy will show grouping of fibres by type, and evidence of denervation and reinnervation. Roussy–Lévy syndrome is similar but patients are aware of a tremor. The lesser types of hereditary motor and sensory neuropathies (types III–VII) are quite rare. The foot disorders are shown in Table 52.1.

3. In later life, patients present with the neurological variant (type II) of the disease. This also has an autosomal dominant inheritance. Although peripheral weakness can be greater, the hands are less often involved. Normal, or near normal, nerve conduction velocities are generally observed on testing and the nerves are not hypertrophic.

4. An orthosis is often required to prevent foot inversion. In mild cases an extended Thomas lateral heel flare on the shoe may suffice, but more severely affected patients will require an ankle-foot orthosis or caliper (Fig. 52.2). A triple arthrodesis is usually necessary eventually to maintain a plantigrade foot. Hand tendon transfers and correction of any scoliosis may also be required in severe cases.

5. Life expectancy should be normal.

Table 52.1 The hereditary motor and sensory neuropathies

Type	Disease	Age	Inheritance	Foot deformity
I	Charcot–Marie–Tooth	<20 years	Dominant	Pes cavus
II	Charcot–Marie–Tooth	Middle age	Dominant	Pes cavus
III	Dejerine–Sottas	Infancy	Recessive	Talipes equinovarus
IV	Refsum	0–30 years	Recessive	Pes cavus. Anomalies of metatarsal length
V		10 years onwards	Recessive	Achilles tendon contracture
VI	+ Optic atrophy		Uncertain	Pes cavus
VII	+ Retinitis pigmentosa		Recessive	Pes cavus

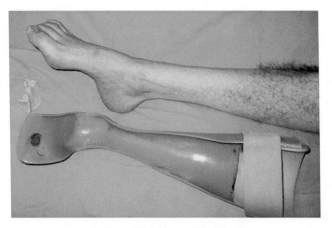

Fig. 52.2 Ankle-foot orthosis

Key points

- There are two common types of hereditary motor and sensory neuropathy with onset at different ages.
- An orthosis is almost always required to prevent foot inversion.
- A triple arthrodesis is frequently necessary in later life.

Further reading

Dyck PJ, Lambert EH (1996) Lower motor and primary sensory neuron diseases with peroneal muscular atrophy. Part I. Neurologic, genetic and electrophysiologic findings in hereditary polyneuropathies. Archives of Neurology 18:603–18.

Dyck PJ, Lambert EH (1996) Lower motor and primary sensory neuron diseases with peroneal muscular atrophy. Part II. Neurologic, genetic, and electrophysiologic findings in various neuronal degenerations. Archives of Neurology 18:619–25.

Guyton GP, Mann RA (2000) The pathogenesis and surgical management of foot deformity in Charcot–Marie–Tooth disease. Foot and Ankle Clinics 5:317–26.

Case 53

Many people have high foot arches yet remain entirely asymptomatic. They only present to podiatry or orthopaedic clinics when they develop clawing of the toes or hard callouses on their soles. In this case a lady in her mid-50s presented to the clinic complaining that she continually walked on the outer border of her foot. A radiograph confirmed that she had marked heel varus (Fig. 53.1).

The lady reported that in 1954 she had surgery to her great toe and the following photographs were retrieved from the hospital archives (Fig. 53.2).

1. What is the likely aetiology of this patient's long-standing cavoid foot?
2. How is the degree of structural deformity quantified?
3. What operations had been performed in 1954?
4. What procedure corrected the hindfoot varus?
5. Is increasing muscle weakness and loss of function typical of patients with this condition in later life?

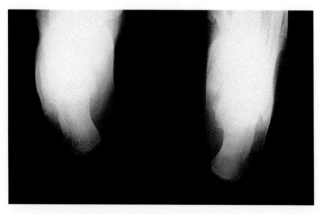

Fig. 53.1 Severe heel varus on standing radiograph

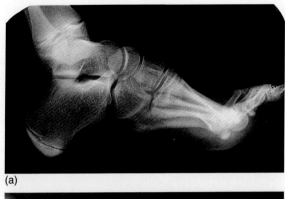

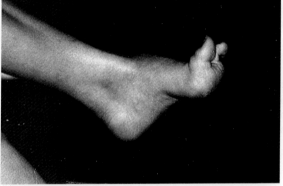

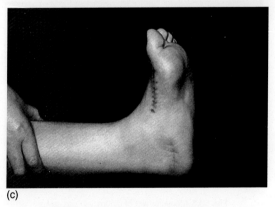

Fig. 53.2 (a–c) Clinical appearance in 1954

Post-polio syndrome

1. In many parts of the world poliomyelitis still remains the most common cause of pes cavus, although similar changes may be evident in patients with cerebral palsy, some forms of muscular dystrophy, Friedreich's ataxia and in hereditary motor sensory neuropathy (Charcot–Marie–Tooth disease; see Fig. 52.1). Muscle imbalance may be extremely subtle yet can lead to significant deformity. In polio there is usually weakness of the dorsiflexor muscles and some calf contracture, although the reverse can occur, leading to calcaneocavus. Frequently, callosities develop under the metatarsal heads, along the outer margin of the foot and across the dorsum of the PIP joints at the site of toe hammering.

2. Pes cavus is quantified by measurement of the first metatarsal-calcaneal angle on a standard weightbearing lateral foot radiograph. This angle will be less than 140°, as in this instance (Fig. 53.3). Although the heel may lie in a neutral position, a structural varus deformity of the forefoot progressively develops with tightening of the plantar fascia. The tendency for the patient to bear weight on the outer border of the foot leads to progressive forefoot adduction.

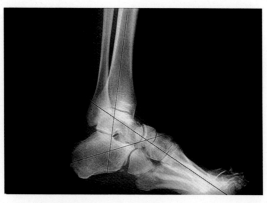

Fig. 53.3 Measurement of deformity in pes cavus

The ultimate aim of surgery for pes cavus is to obtain a plantigrade foot. If the tibioplantar angle exceeds 120°, then forefoot cavus will not be corrected by a basal metatarsal or tarsometatarsal wedge excision without creating a rocker bottom foot and a triple arthrodesis is generally required.

3. At the age of 11 years, this patient had a Steindler release of the plantar fascia from her heel, with a 70% correction of the cavus. Subsequently, extensor hallucis longus was transferred to the neck of the first metatarsal (Jones transfer). The surgeon chose not to fuse the IP joint of the great toe. Tibialis anterior function was noted to be strong and further surgery, such as transfer of extensor digitorum longus tendons to the cuneiforms (Hibbs procedure), was not required.

4. The primary residual deformity at the patient's recent presentation was the severe varus of her heel on her left side. She had no subtalar pain and a lateral closing wedge osteotomy of the calcaneus (Dwyer's osteotomy) produced an extremely satisfactory end result (Fig. 53.4).

   In this case the patient's forefoot cavus was not especially severe and a more distal dorsal tarsal wedge osteotomy (or Japas' V osteotomy) was not required.

5. Post-polio syndrome is the onset of new neurological manifestations that occur in patients 10–40 years after recovery from acute polio. It is characterized by fatigue, weakness, joint and muscle pain and worsening functional abilities.

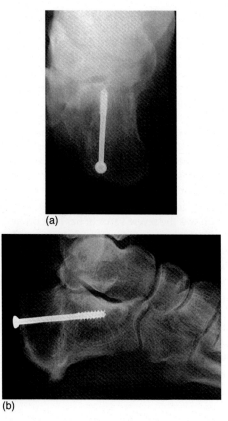

Fig 53.4 (a, b) Correction of heel varus by lateral closing wedge osteotomy

Key points

- Pes cavus is common and is frequently asymptomatic.
- Surgery should be undertaken in the teenage years if possible.
- A calcaneal osteotomy will be required to correct heel varus.
- Progressive muscle weakness may be part of a 'post-polio syndrome'.

Further reading

Dwyer FC (1959) Osteotomy of the calcaneum for pes cavus. Journal of Bone and Joint Surgery 41-B:80–6.

Howard RS (2007) Poliomyelitis and the postpolio syndrome. British Medical Journal 330:1314–18.

Japas LM (1968) Surgical treatment of pes cavus by tarsal V-osteotomy: preliminary report. Journal of Bone and Joint Surgery 50-A:927–44.

Schwend RM, Drennan JC (2003) Cavus foot deformity in children. Journal of the American Academy of Orthopaedic Surgeons 11:201–11.

Section 8

Trauma

Case 54

A 36-year-old window cleaner presents, having slipped 20 feet off a ladder. He landed awkwardly on his left heel, which immediately became extremely swollen. In casualty a radiograph confirmed that he had fractured his calcaneus (Fig. 54.1).

1. What is the most common mechanism of injury and what other fractures might have been sustained when the patient fell?
2. How are calcaneal fractures classified? What methods might be used to ascertain the exact type of injury?
3. What treatment is appropriate for this patient?
4. Will the long-term prognosis be favourable?

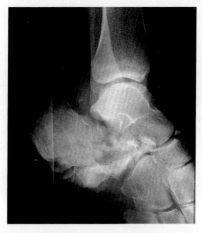

Fig. 54.1 Fracture of calcaneus

Fracture of the calcaneus

1. Most frequently patients land on a pronated foot, destroying their medial longitudinal arch and forcing the heel into valgus. The peroneal tendons will generally be held in their groove on an intact lateral wall. Vertical shear force will produce an initial fracture line (described by Palmer; Fig. 54.2), splitting the bone into two parts: an anteromedial fragment including the sustentaculum tali and a posterolateral fragment including the calcaneal tuberosity. Further fractures propagate according to the force and exact direction of injury.

   Calcaneal fractures are bilateral in 5–10% of patients, associated with other lower limb fractures in up to 25% and with a lumbar spinal fracture in 10%.

2. In terms of future disability, fractures with an intra-articular extension will generally have a poorer prognosis than those that do not. Calcaneal fractures are no exception and early radiological classifications (by Böhler and Essex-Lopresti) subdivided the fracture types into two primary groups, according to whether the posterior subtalar articular surface was involved.

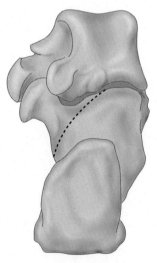

Fig. 54.2 Primary vertical shear fracture

Extra-articular fractures (25% of the total) of the upper or lower border of the body, tuberosity, anterior process and sustentaculum tali generally have a good clinical prognosis, with many patients able to return to work within 6 months.

Transarticular fractures are less easily classified. Essex-Lopresti considered two primary subgroups. In the first type a downward force causes heel eversion at the subtalar joint and a 'tongue-type' fracture (Fig. 54.3). In the second, a shear force typically fractures off the sustentaculum tali, depressing the centrolateral articular segment into the calcaneal body, as shown in

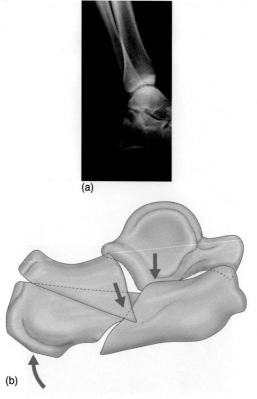

(a)

(b)

Fig. 54.3 (a, b) Tongue-type fracture

Figures 54.1 and 54.4. This classification was further refined by Sanders et al in 1990 based on the number and location of the articular fracture fragments on a coronal CT (Fig. 54.5).

3. Heel fractures are invariably accompanied by massive soft tissue contusion, and immediate high elevation of the injured foot is essential (Fig. 54.6). In this case, the patient's fracture was also extremely comminuted and it was felt that the joint surface was destroyed beyond salvage. However, as noted on the CT image, the heel was excessively splayed. A closed manipulation was performed under general anaesthetic, once the initial swelling was down, and a well-padded plaster cast applied. After a further period as an inpatient with his foot elevated, the patient was

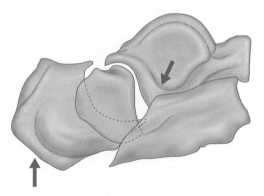

Fig. 54.4 Joint depression fracture

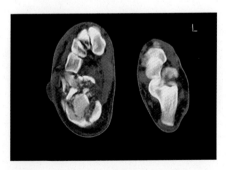

Fig. 54.5 Coronal CT scans showing severe comminution and primary shear

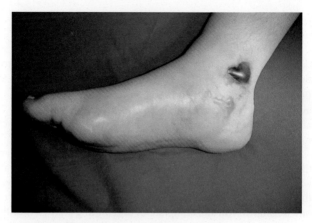

Fig. 54.6 Inner sole bruising (Oxford sign) with fracture blistering

allowed to mobilize on crutches without weightbearing. The cast was retained for 6 weeks. Despite intensive physiotherapy during the next 3 months the joint progressively ankylosed (Fig. 54.7).

If surgery had been possible, then the essence of treatment would have been to realign the subtalar joint, restoring Böhler's calcaneal-tuber joint angle (the angle between the superior surfaces of the calcaneus) to that of the opposite foot (normal range 25–40°). A tongue-type fracture may simply be displaced back into position using a lever, sometimes termed a Gissane

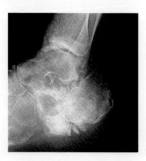

Fig. 54.7 Subtalar joint destruction

spike, inserted posteriorly into the bone. The fracture can be held with a couple of screws or staples (Fig. 54.8).

Open reduction and fixation is generally required for joint depression fractures. Often bone grafts must be inserted to buttress the joint and the fracture is then usually held by a plate (Fig. 54.9).

4. Rehabilitation after a calcaneal fracture is prolonged and the average time off work for patients in most reported series is about 6 months. Function is impaired by any ankle, subtalar or midtarsal joint stiffness.

Heel cushioning may help relieve pain caused by disruption of the heel fat pad, but if bone spurs on the sole or lateral calcaneal wall cause localized pressure or tendon impingement respectively, then bone resection may be necessary. A few patients, such as the one illustrated, will still complain of unremitting pain 12 months after injury. A formal subtalar fusion may then be the only option.

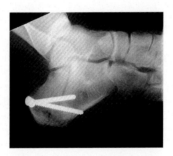

Fig. 54.8 Fracture stabilization with interfragmentary screws

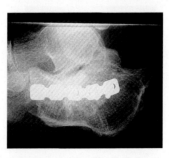

Fig. 54.9 Lateral wall buttress plate

Evidence

Four trials were included in the Cochrane Collaborative review (Bridgman et al 1999) of interventions for calcaneal fractures but all had methodological flaws. Three trials, involving 134 patients, compared open reduction and internal fixation with non-operative management of displaced intra-articular fractures. Pooled results showed no differences in residual pain 12–15 months after treatment between the groups, but after surgery, more patients were able to return to work and wear the same shoes as before their trauma. One very small trial suggested that impulse compression therapy may be beneficial. Two more recent randomized controlled trials produced conflicting results on the benefits of surgery.

Key points

- Bruising on the inner aspect of the sole suggests a heel fracture: 'the Oxford sign'.
- High elevation of the foot will lessen initial discomfort.
- Restoration of subtalar joint congruity is the key to a good clinical outcome.
- Bone grafting may be required to buttress the joint surface.
- Physiotherapy is essential to prevent stiffness.

Further reading

Bridgman SA, Dunn KM, McBride DJ, Richards PJ (1999) Interventions for treating calcaneal fractures. Cochrane Database of Systematic Reviews, Issue 4.

Essex-Lopresti P (1952) The mechanism, reduction technique and results in fractures of the os calcis. British Journal of Surgery 39:395–419.

Magnan B, Bortolazzi R, Marangon A, Marino M, Dall'Oca C, Bartolozzi P (2006) External fixation for displaced intra-articular fractures of the calcaneum. Journal of Bone and Joint Surgery 88-B:1474–9.

Sanders R (2000) Current concepts review – displaced intra-articular fractures of the calcaneus. Journal of Bone and Joint Surgery 82:225–50.

Stephenson JR (1987) Treatment of displaced intra-articular fractures of the calcaneus using medial and lateral approaches, internal fixation and early motion. Journal of Bone and Joint Surgery 69-A:115–30.

Case 55

Despite braking as hard as possible, a 22-year-old student was unable to prevent his Alfa Romeo crashing at speed into an oncoming car. He suffered the compound fracture shown in Figure 55.1.

1. What exactly has caused this injury?
2. Who described these injuries and what type would this be?
3. Is subchondral bone atrophy significant? When is avascular necrosis likely to be evident?
4. Would there be merit in any form of hindfoot arthrodesis? If so, which and when?

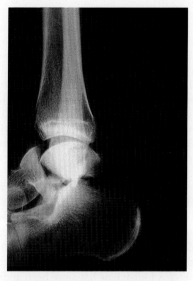

Fig. 55.1 Compound fracture of hindfoot

1. It was always assumed that talar neck fractures were caused by the leading edge of the tibia striking the talus when the foot was excessively and forcibly dorsiflexed. Cadaveric modelling, however, suggests that it is more likely that it is simply the midfoot which is hyperextended on the talus, when the leg and foot are outstretched, i.e. the hindfoot is held rigid by a taut Achilles tendon. Such a position typically occurs in a 'head-on' motor vehicle accident when the foot is pushed upwards by the pedals or, as originally described, by a similar mechanism in a light aircraft crash, 'the aviator's fracture'. Recently, a boy of 9 years was admitted after sledging backwards (Fig. 55.2).

2. Hawkins classified injuries of the talar neck into three groups: type I, undisplaced talar neck fracture; type II, fracture of the talus with subluxation of the subtalar joint; type III, fracture of the talus with dislocation of the bone from both the subtalar and ankle joints. A fourth type has since been added to take into account any associated subluxation or dislocation of the talar head off the navicular bone.

    The 22-year-old patient described suffered a type II injury. He was treated by wound debridement and stabilization of the fracture with two lagged cortical screws (Fig. 55.3).

3. Although fracture malunion can occur, leading to impingement of the dorsal bone surface on the margin of the distal tibia on dorsiflexion, we have found that the protuberant lip of bone is generally resectable and patients regain normal foot function. In stark contrast, avascular necrosis develops slowly and it may be up to 2 years before the condition becomes clinically evident. Avascular necrosis occurs in up to 50% of type II injuries, however treated. Subchondral bone atrophy (Hawkins' sign), seen approximately 6 weeks after a talar fracture is said to be a good prognostic indicator. The sign is probably a reflection of increased localized bone vascularity and healing (Fig. 55.4).

4. Once avascular necrosis sets in, or if there is significant articular damage to either the subtalar or ankle joints, then further surgery is generally required. Unfortunately, the loss of talar height will mitigate against a successful single joint arthrodesis. Pantalar hindfoot arthrodesis may be the only viable option and

some leg length discrepancy from shortening is an inevitable result. Most trauma surgeons would not consider astragalectomy (talus excision).

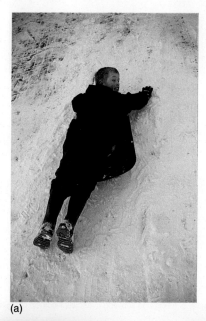
(a)

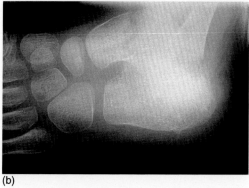
(b)

Fig. 55.2 (a, b) Talar neck fracture in a sledger

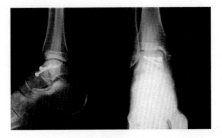

Fig. 55.3 Talar neck fracture held by screws

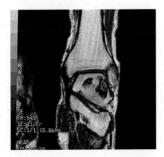

Fig. 55.4 MR image showing avascular necrosis of talus

Key points

- Talar neck fractures were classified by Hawkins.
- Avascular necrosis may not be evident for up to 2 years.
- Hawkins' sign indicates a favourable prognosis.

Further reading

Hawkins L (1970) Fractures of the neck of the talus. Journal of Bone and Joint Surgery 52-A:991–1002.

Lindvall E, Haidukewych G, DiPasquale T, Herscovici D, Sanders R (2004) Open reduction and stable fixation of isolated, displaced talar neck and body fractures. Journal of Bone and Joint Surgery 86-A:2229–34.

Metzger MJ, Levin JS, Clancy JT (1999) Talar neck fractures and rates of avascular necrosis. Journal of Foot and Ankle Surgery 38:154–62.

Case 56

This 58-year-old women presents with a 6-week history of dull aching pain in the forefoot experienced on prolonged weight-bearing; she denies any injury to her foot. She is diffusely tender across her forefoot and there is a tender swelling over her metatarsals. An AP radiograph is shown in Figure 56.1.

1. What is her diagnosis and what is the cause of this 'injury'?
2. What are the risk factors for this condition in middle-aged women?
3. How should her injury be treated?
4. Why are radiographs of limited value in the diagnosis of this condition?
5. What other investigation(s) can be used?

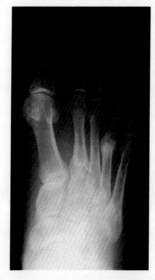

Fig. 56.1 AP radiograph of foot

Stress fracture of metatarsals

1. She has suffered stress fractures of the neck of her fourth metatarsal and base of second metatarsal. Stress fractures occur in normal bones subjected to forces occurring for a prolonged or repeated period. The force are insufficient to cause an acute fracture. In sedentary individuals, the cause is usually related to unaccustomed activity. Classically, the patient was an army recruit with the stress fracture being induced by strenuous square bashing or route marching ('march' fracture). Stress fractures of the metatarsals can also be seen in highly trained athletes through 'overuse'.

2. Postmenopausal osteopenia will make a metatarsal more susceptible to fracture (insufficiency fracture). Radiographs do not show obvious osteopenia. In this case a dual energy X-ray absorptiometry (DEXA) scan was performed and this was found to be normal, ruling out osteoporosis.

3. Immobilization was indicated to alleviate pain and encourage bone healing. This was provided in the form of a 'moon boot' (Fig. 56.2) and the patient advised to use crutches. At follow-up 6 weeks later, her pain had improved but a radiograph showed delayed union of the fracture at the base of the second metatarsal (Fig. 56.3).

4. Radiographs have limited value because initially they often appear normal. Dorsoplantar views are the most useful but an oblique view is also recommended. Radiographic evidence of the fracture does not take place until 3 weeks after injury when endosteal and periosteal bone callus becomes evident. For example, Figure 56.4a shows a normal radiograph of a young girl seen in A&E with a painful foot. Her metatarsal stress fracture was not confirmed until some weeks later by repeat radiography (Fig. 56.4b).

   In the absence of immediate radiological evidence it should be assumed that a patient has suffered a stress fracture when there is a clear-cut clinical history. Follow-up radiographs are required to confirm bony union with significant callus formation.

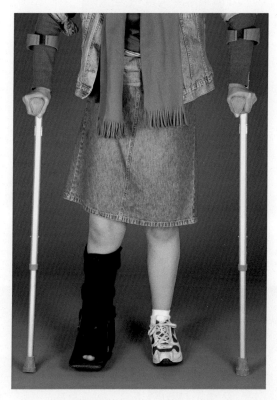

Fig. 56.2 Moon boot and double crutches

5. Radio-isotope bone scans (scintigraphs) utilizing technetium phosphate 99mTc (half-life 6 hours) detects metabolic bone changes within 24 hours. In case 56, a CT scan (Fig. 56.5) was requested and the patient was instructed to persist with her moon boot. Despite this, the fracture failed to unite but, as she was now asymptomatic, she declined open reduction and internal fixation.

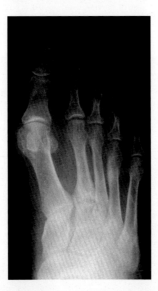

Fig. 56.3 Review X-ray shows healing of fourth metatarsal fracture and a hypertrophic non-union of the second metatarsal base

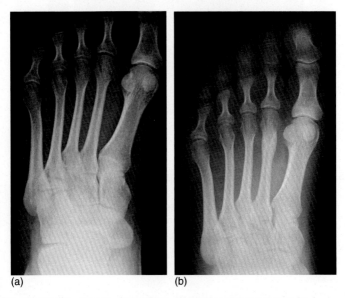

(a)   (b)

Fig. 56.4 (a) AP radiograph at time of injury. (b) Repeat radiograph 6 weeks later showing callus formation at the neck of the second metatarsal

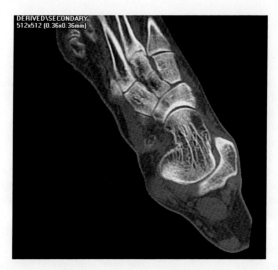

Fig. 56.5 CT scan showing hypertrophic non-union of second metatarsal fracture

Key points

- Stress fractures occur in normal bones subjected to normal forces occurring for a prolonged or repeated period.
- Initial radiographs are often normal. Fractures are not evident until bone healing has been established, up to 6 weeks following initial injury
- Postmenopausal osteopenia will make a metatarsal more susceptible to fracture (insufficiency fracture).
- Treatment is by immobilization with a trauma shoe (forefoot off-loading), moon boot or sometimes a plaster of Paris cast.
- Non-united metatarsal fractures do not always require intervention.

Further reading

Petrisor BA, Ekrol I, Court-Brown C (2006) The epidemiology of metatarsal fractures. Foot and Ankle International 27(3):172–4.

Case 57

A 60-year-old lady presented to A&E complaining that she had slipped on a stairway in a shopping mall. She complained of an extremely sore left heel. The Casualty Officer found that she retained a full range of ankle movement but that she was unable to stand on her toes. An X-ray of her ankle was normal.

An ankle sprain was diagnosed and the patient's ankle was immobilized in a short-leg weight-bearing plaster. The cast was removed 2 weeks later.

The lady's pain persisted throughout the next 3 months. She finally sought a further opinion from her GP who found a lump at the insertion of her Achilles tendon. Surgical exploration revealed what is shown in Figure 57.1

1. What clinical test should the Casualty Officer have performed?
2. If the diagnosis had been correctly made, would plaster immobilization of the ankle have been appropriate treatment?
3. How can a chronically ruptured tendon be reconstituted and what complications may arise?

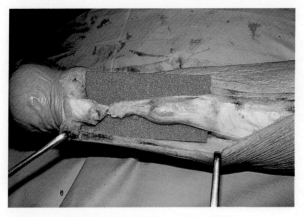

Fig. 57.1 Chronic rupture of Achilles tendon

Chronic rupture of Achilles tendon

1. Simmonds' (or Thompson's) test is performed with the patient kneeling on the side of an examination couch. Absence of plantarflexion of the left foot, as shown when this patient was examined, indicated that her Achilles tendon was ruptured (Fig. 57.2).

2. In young patients, in whom one would expect good healing, conservative treatment is reasonable (see Evidence below). Ideally, the foot should be immobilized in full equinus for 4 weeks, semi-equinus for 4 weeks and then in a 90° cast for a further fortnight. The patient is then encouraged to wear a shoe with a 2 cm heel raise for a further 3 months. An alternative is to place the patient into a functional brace at 6 weeks for 6 weeks (Fig. 57.3).

   In this case, the patient was slightly older than average and if an early diagnosis had been made, then either an open or semi-open (percutaneous) repair method would have been appropriate. Some surgeons recommend the use of implantable polyester tapes.

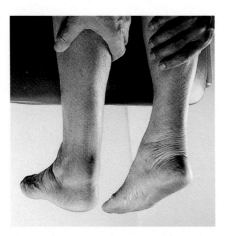

Fig. 57.2 Simmonds' test for Achilles tendon rupture (positive on left)

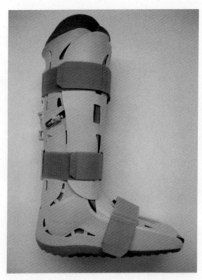

Fig. 57.3 Functional Aircast® brace

3. If a tear is long-standing, the tendon ends cannot easily be approximated and some form of tendon augmentation is required. Our preference is to slide the tendon distally by a V-Y plasty at the musculotendinous junction (Fig. 57.4) or, if some tissue can be stretched across the gap, to use flexor hallucis longus (FHL) tendon as an active augment (Fig. 57.5). Tendon atrophy may occur, with subsequent wound breakdown, when either plantaris or a long strip of the median raphe of gastrocnemius has been turned down across the gap, as shown in Figure 57.6. Presumably this is because the tendon slip is virtually avascular. Subsequent wound salvage may require sophisticated plastic surgery using either a fascial flap or a microvascular free flap, transferred from the forearm or anterolateral thigh.

This patient still had persistent pain and discomfort at her heel 9 months after surgery, with some residual calf muscle weakness. This is not an uncommon finding even if a ruptured tendon is treated acutely.

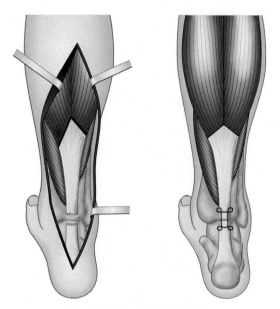

Fig. 57.4 Myofascial slide (V-Y plasty)

Evidence

Data from 800 patients were reported from 12 randomized controlled trials (Khan et al 2005) comparing treatments of acute Achilles tendon ruptures. The rate of re-rupture was lower in the operatively treated group than in the non-operative group (3.5% versus 12.6%), but the complication rate was higher (34.1% versus 2.7%). The re-rupture rates of open and percutaneous methods were respectively 4.3% and 2.1% and complication rates 26.1% and 8.3%, favouring the minimally invasive technique. Following surgery, the rate of re-rupture was 50% less when functional bracing followed cast immobilization as compared with cast immobilization alone. This difference was even more marked in the non-operative group.

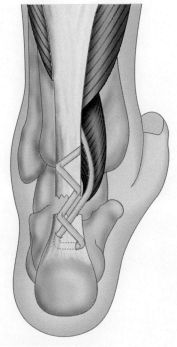

Fig. 57.5 Flexor hallucis longus augment (the distal end of FHL is sutured to flexor digitorum longus)

Key points

- Achilles tendon rupture is most likely with oblique loading (for example, on heel adduction) of a maximally contracted muscle.
- Conservative management may lead to slower restoration of normal function but postoperative complications are avoided.
- Repair of a chronic rupture generally requires tendon augmentation. A myofascial slide is recommended.

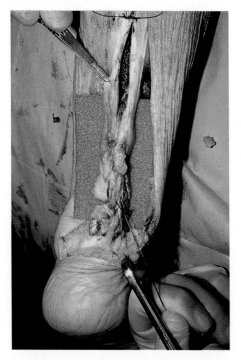

Fig. 57.6 Bosworth repair of Achilles tendon (not recommended)

Further reading

Khan RJK, Fick D, Keogh A, Crawford J, Brammar T, Parker M (2005) Treatment of acute Achilles tendon rupture. A meta-analysis of randomised controlled trials. Journal of Bone and Joint Surgery 87-A:2202–10.

Maffulli N, Ajis A (2008) Management of chronic ruptures of the Achilles tendon. Journal of Bone and Joint Surgery 90-A:1348–60.

Wapner KL, Hecht PJ, Mills RH (1995) Reconstruction of neglected Achilles tendon injury. Orthopedic Clinics of North America 26:249–63.

Webb JM, Bannister GC (1999) Percutaneous repair of the ruptured tendon Achillis. Journal of Bone and Joint Surgery 81-B:877–80.

Case 58

An overweight, 65-year-old lady reports a constant ache in her foot arches, extending into her calf. She was also aware of an event in which her feet 'gave way' and her 'arches dropped'. Since this event her ache has lessened but she now complains of a weakness in her feet and a lack of spring in her step. This patient has also noted that she now needs a larger size of shoes (Fig. 58.1).

1. What is the most likely diagnosis for this patient's complaint?
2. Explain why she now requires a larger shoe size?
3. Which striking clinical feature is exhibited in Figure 58.1?
4. What further clinical examination should be carried out?
5. How does the type of dysfunction relate to treatment?

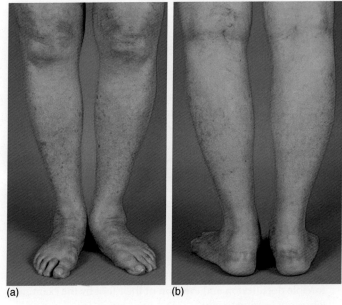

Fig. 58.1 (a, b) Clinical appearance of patient's feet – frontal and posterior views

Tibialis posterior rupture

1. Posterior tibial tendon rupture is the most likely diagnosis. It is a degenerative disorder seen predominantly in elderly females with pes planovalgus.

2. Patients may report an increase in shoe size as the feet excessively pronate and consequently elongate.

3. The 'too many toes' sign which occurs with excessive foot pronation results in abduction of the forefoot on the hindfoot.

4. Further examination requires the patient to stand on one foot and then tiptoe. Most patients with a rupture of the tibialis posterior tendon will find this difficult, although it is still possible with the aid of the other posterior calf muscles. To distinguish tibialis posterior dysfunction, the test should be taken a step further and the patient asked to transfer their weight from the outside of their foot to the inside. Dysfunction of the tendon is apparent when the patient fails to perform this action, instead swaying at the hips in an attempt to transfer load on the foot. The patient will also be unable to counteract forcible dorsiflexion and eversion of their foot by the examiner, when not bearing weight.

5. Several stages of tendon dysfunction are recognized and the treatment is dependent upon the exact pathology (Table 58.1). Direct repair of a recently ruptured tendon may be possible, but a graft will usually be required if the tear is long-standing. Most commonly, flexor digitorum longus is surgically divided and the proximal end attached to the distal stump of tibialis posterior. The distal end of flexor digitorum longus may then be joined to flexor hallucis longus, although flexion of the lesser toes is actually still possible through the action of flexor digitorum brevis and the lumbrical muscles. Unfortunately, many patients are seen far too late even for such a reconstruction. The presence of hindfoot arthritis will mitigate against success and the only surgical solution is then a triple arthrodesis to correct the hindfoot malalignment.

   If the patient is unfit for surgery, her footwear should be modified to prevent hindfoot pronation. Simplest is probably the addition of a medial heel flare (Fig. 58.2), but a Thomas-style heel will also help if coupled with a supportive in-shoe wedge.

Table 58.1 Classification of tibialis posterior dysfunction

Stage	Signs	Treatment
I Tenosynovitis without deformity A: Inflammatory B: Partial with normal hindfoot C: Partial with hindfoot valgus	Minimal deformity Intact single leg heel raise	Tenosynovectomy plus a medial calcaneal osteotomy if any hindfoot valgus
II Ruptured tibialis posterior with flexible flat foot A: Hindfoot valgus B: Flexible forefoot supination C: Fixed forefoot supination D: Forefoot abduction E: Medial ray instability	Heel will reduce from valgus position but variable associated forefoot deformity	Transfer of flexor digitorum longus and medial translational osteotomy of the calcaneus. If forefoot supination then gastrocnemius recession (flexible) or opening wedge osteotomy of medial cuneiform (fixed). If forefoot abducted then lateral column lengthening osteotomy of os calcis. Address medial ray instability by arthrodesis of tarsometatarsal joint
III Rigid hindfoot valgus A: Hindfoot valgus B: Transverse tarsal abduction	Rigidity of hindfoot Rigidity of abducted forefoot	Triple arthodesis plus bone block lengthening of calcaneocuboid joint if tarsal abduction
IV Ankle valgus A: Flexible ankle valgus B: Rigid ankle valgus	Medial ankle instability	As stage II or III with deltoid ligament reconstruction (flexible) or ankle arthrodesis (rigid)

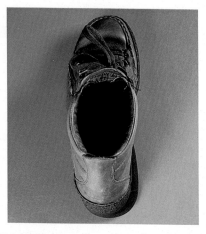

Fig. 58.2 Medial shoe heel flare for tibialis posterior dysfunction

Key points

- Tibialis posterior dysfunction is generally seen as a degenerative disorder.
- Patients are typically elderly overweight women.
- Orthoses are designed to prevent foot pronation.
- Surgery is an option for acute injuries.

Further reading

Holmes GB, Mann RA (1992) Possible etiological factors associated with rupture of the posterior tibial tendon. Foot and Ankle International 13:70–9.

Johnson KA, Strom DE (1989) Tibialis posterior tendon dysfunction. Clinical Orthopedics 239:196–206.

Mosier SM, Lucas DR, Pomeroy G, Manoli A (1998) Pathology of the posterior tibial tendon in posterior tibial tendon insufficiency. Foot and Ankle International 19:520–4.

Myerson MS, Badekas A, Shcon LC (2004) Treatment of stage II posterior tibial tendon deficiency with flexor digitorum longus tendon transfer and calcaneal osteotomy. Foot and Ankle International 25:445–50.

Zwipp H, Rammelt S (2006) Modified Evans osteotomy for the operative treatment of acquired pes planovalgus. Operative Orthopadie und Traumatologie 18:182–97.

Case 59

A 35-year-old woman jumped down approximately 2 metres off a wall while out hill-walking. She was subsequently brought to Casualty where she was found to have an extremely bruised forefoot. The radiograph is shown opposite (Fig. 59.1).

1. What injury is this?
2. What is the mechanism of trauma and how are these dislocations classified?
3. What is the key to fracture reduction and stability?
4. Can a reasonable functional result be expected?

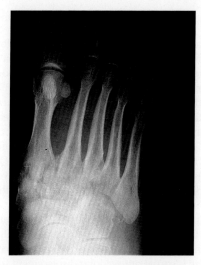

Fig. 59.1 Right foot following injury

1. The radiograph shows a fracture dislocation of the forefoot through Lisfranc's joint. Lisfranc (1790–1847) was a French surgeon of renown who was best known for his work on rectal cancer. His name has been accorded to the ligament anchoring the base of the second metatarsal to the medial cuneiform. This ligament effectively holds the base of the second metatarsal into its recess between the cuneiforms. There is no ligament between the first and second metatarsal bases. Various modifications of an early classification of fracture dislocations by Quénu & Kuss (1909) have been put forward. Most were derived from a consideration of the direction of imparted force to the forefoot. In the coronal plane, there may be total incongruity of the joint (a), a partial displacement with only part of the joint incongruent following a lateral (b) or medial force (c) and, finally, the result of a divergent force that may again be subdivided according to whether there is partial or total joint displacement (d), as shown in Figure 59.2.

    Lisfranc injuries may also be classified into those of high and low energy. In a high-speed road accident it is common for the driver to fix his or her foot fimly on the brake pedal to resist forward motion after impact. This causes a direct force pushing the tarsus (45%) or metatarsals (55%) in a volar direction. Athletes usually suffer injuries of low velocity, sustained (95%) when falling backwards on a plantarflexed foot, for example during windsurfing or horseriding, with dorsal displacement of the metatarsals.

2. The key to reduction is the placement of the base of the second metatarsal back into its recess. It may be possible to manage this by closed reduction under general anaesthesia, but often the reduction will not be stable and fixation using multiple K-wires or screws is required (Fig. 59.3). The tibialis anterior tendon may become trapped between the medial and intermediate cuneiform bones, blocking reduction of the first metatarsal. Open reduction is then essential. Care should be taken that local bleeding and general contusion of the soft tissues have not led to a dorsal foot compartment syndrome. It is generally advisable to release any fascia that appears excessively tight. Patients are kept non-weightbearing for 6 weeks following

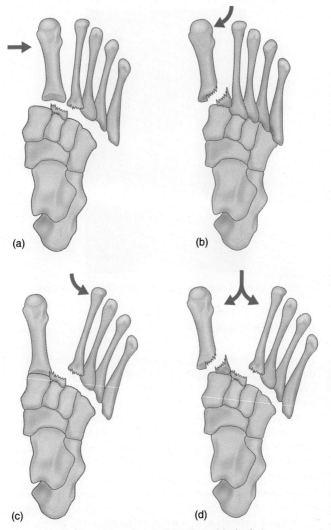

Fig. 59.2 Lisfranc fracture dislocations of the forefoot

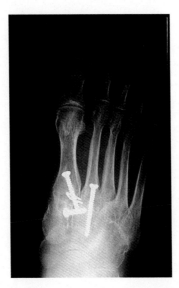

Fig. 59.3 Lisfranc dislocation stabilized with interfragmentary screws

surgery, then mobilized agressively to prevent reflex sympathetic dystrophy.

3. The outcome is very much dependent on accurate diagnosis and treatment. Care should be taken in patients with multiple injuries to ensure that a Lisfranc dislocation is not missed. Initially, the only sign present may be a bruising under the skin of the midfoot (Lisfranc's sign). It is only later, when weightbearing, that a 'gap' indicative of divergence of the first and second metatarsals becomes evident. Patients may not provide a history of acute trauma, as the deformity can be the end result of repetitive injury, especially if a patient has peripheral neuropathy.

4. Unfortunately, even with expeditious treatment, patients often complain of long-term pain in the forefoot. As seen in Figure 59.1, many patients have fractures extending into at least one of the midfoot joints and the end result may be progressive osteoarthritis and residual joint displacement. Most patients will end up with a flat foot deformity and walk with an increased load on their hindfoot.

Evidence

Primary stable arthrodesis of the medial two or three rays was shown by Thuan & Coetzee (2006) to be better than internal fixation for ligamentous injuries in one trial with alternate assignment. Data from one other RCT suggest that complete arthrodesis for severe Lisfranc injuries should be avoided and that only the medial two or three rays should be fused.

Key points

- Lisfranc dislocation may be missed – look for plantar bruising.
- The base of the second metatarsal must sit in its recess.
- Stabilization is generally required.
- Long-term stiffness is common.

Further reading

Buzzard BM, Briggs PJ (1998) Surgical management of acute tarsometatarsal fracture dislocation in the adult. Clinical Orthopedics 353:125–33.

Hardcastle PH, Reschauer R, Kutscha-Lissberg E, Schoffmann W (1982) Injuries to the tarsometatarsal joint. Incidence, classification and treatment. Journal of Bone and Joint Surgery 64-B:349–56.

Mulier T, Reynders P, Dereymaeker G, Broos P (2002) Severe Lisfranc injuries: primary arthrodesis or ORIF? Foot and Ankle International 23:902–5.

Thuan VL, Coetzee JC (2006) Treatment of primarily ligamentous Lisfranc joint injuries: primary arthrodesis compared with open reduction and internal fixation. Journal of Bone and Joint Surgery 88-A:514–20.

Case 60

A 40-year-old hill-walker presents to the clinic complaining that his ankle aches when he descends all but the flattest of slopes. New lightweight boots did not make the slightest difference to his symptoms. The radiograph is shown in Figure 60.1.

1. What is the natural history of this talar lesion?
2. How might the lesion be further assessed?
4. Is surgical treatment ever of value?

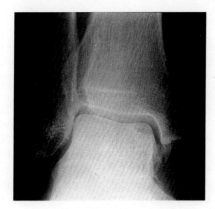

Fig. 60.1 AP ankle radiograph

Osteochondral lesions of the talus

1. Osteochondritis of the talus is generally initiated by direct
    trauma to the ankle. It is very similar in many respects
    to osteochondritis dissecans in the knee. The following
    radiographic classification is commonly used.

    Stage I: A small area of compression of the subchondral
               bone. The articular cartilage remains intact.

    Stage II: A partially detached osteochondral fragment. The
               anterior talofibular and calcaneofibular ligaments
               will have ruptured.

    Stage III: A completely detatched fragment that remains in its
               talar crater.

    Stage IV: A displaced fragment.

    The fractures occur with a similar frequency on the
    medial and lateral borders of the talus. The lateral lesions
    are generally located in the middle third of the talar margin,
    as during inversion of a dorsiflexed ankle the talus rotates
    laterally in the frontal plane, causing impingement of its
    margin against the fibula. In contrast, medial lesions, caused
    when an inversion force is placed on a plantarflexed ankle, are
    sited further posteriorly at the point of impingement of the
    talar dome.

2. The exact nature of the lesion may be assessed by plain X-ray,
    tomography, CT scanning, MR imaging, or arthroscopically.
    Chronic lesions may develop a sclerotic margin to the bone
    surrounding the lesion (low intensity on T1-weighted MRI).

3. The aim of treatment is to offload the talar lesion, thus
    reducing pain, improving joint function and in the long
    term limiting joint degeneration. Symptomatic relief may
    be gained from wearing either a medial or lateral heel flare,
    depending on the site of the lesion, but repair of the defect
    will require surgical intervention. Arthroscopic drilling
    into the subchondral plate below the lesion may stimulate
    neovascularization and healing. This will only be appropriate
    for young patients with mild sclerosis of the talar bone
    around the defect, continuity of the cartilaginous surface and
    stability of the fragment. A hinged fragment will have to be
    stabilized, using small pins or screws, or, if detached, then

removed (grades III and IV). Subsequently any defect can be repaired by either osteocartilaginous grafting using block or multiple core grafts, harvested from a non-weightbearing area of the knee (mosaicplasty; Fig. 60.2c), or by autologous

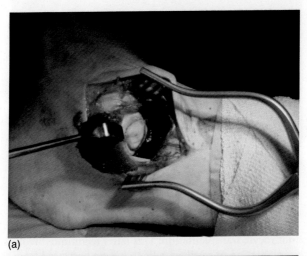

(a)

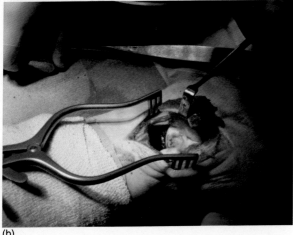

(b)

Fig. 60.2 (a) Osteochondral defect exposed by medial malleolar osteotomy. (b) Osteochondral defect with flap turned back.

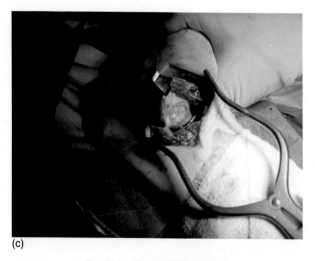

(c)

Fig. 60.2 — Cont'd (c) Mosaicplasty

chondrocyte transplantation. This latter technique involves reimplantation of cartilage cells that were harvested from the anterior talus and subsequently cultured in serum.

Key points

- Talar osteochondritis generally follows forced ankle inversion.
- MRI is useful to determine if the fragment remains attached.
- A heel flare may be beneficial.
- Defects may be repaired by osteocartilaginous grafting or autologous chondrocyte transplantation.

Further reading

Baums MH, Heidrich G, Schultz W, Steckel H, Kahl E, Klinger HM (2006) Autologous chondrocyte transplantation for treating cartilage defects of the talus. Journal of Bone and Joint Surgery 88-A:303–8.

Giannini S, Buda R, Faldini C et al (2005) Surgical treatment of osteochondral lesions of the talus in young active patients. Journal of Bone and Joint Surgery 87-A (suppl 2):28–41.

Hangody L, Kish G, Modis L, Szerb I, Gaspar L, Dioszegi Z, Kendik Z (2001) Mosaicplasty for the treatment of osteochondritis dissecans of the talus: two to seven year results in 36 patients. Foot and Ankle International 22:552–8.

Section 9

Sports injuries

Case 61

A 32-year-old rugby union player sustained an injury to his ankle when his foot was forced inwardly during a ruck (Fig. 61.1). For some time, he has been aware of his ankle giving way when walking. A radiograph was requested (Fig. 61.2).

1. What does the radiograph show?
2. What are the components of the lateral ankle ligament? How do these contribute to joint stability?
3. How might the rugby player's joint instability be addressed?
4. When should he be allowed to mobilise following surgery?

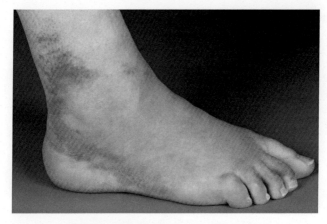

Fig. 61.1 Bruising lateral side rugby player's ankle

Lateral ankle ligament laxity

1. Stress views, with the ankle fully inverted, in this man revealed talar tilting (Fig. 61.2a). In one study, MRI was found to have no distinct advantage over examination under anaesthesia and stress radiography in the diagnosis of severe ligament injuries.

2. Inversion of the talus is prevented when the ankle is plantar flexed by the anterior talofibular ligament (ATFL) and when dorsiflexed by the calcaneofibular ligament (CFL). If the CFL is torn then the ATFL is usually always torn as well. The posterior talofibular ligament and the lateral talocalcaneal ligament are less important with respect to stability of the joint.

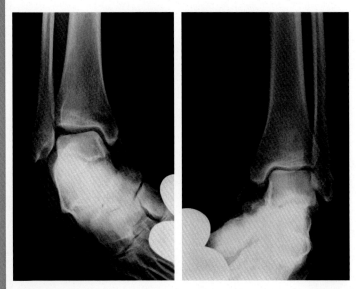

Fig. 61.2 (a) Stress x-ray right ankle showing talar tilting. (b) Stress x-ray of normal left ankle

3. Non-operative treatment should be directed at strengthening up the peroneal muscles by concentric and eccentric exercises to try and improve muscle balance and joint control.

   In 1966, Bröstrom reported on direct late repair of the ankle ligaments. Essentially the torn ends of ATFL (Fig. 61.3) are approximated (Fig. 61.4) with overlap as necessary. Anchoring sutures may be helpful. After repair of the ATFL and CFL it may be possible to re-attach the margin of the extensor retinaculum to the distal fibula as shown in Figure 61.5.

   If there is any residual laxity of the joint following direct anatomical reconstruction then the repair is generally augmented by a graft. Most commonly, part or all of peroneus brevis is detached proximally, then threaded through the fibula as described by Evans (Fig 61.6) and Chrisman-Snook.

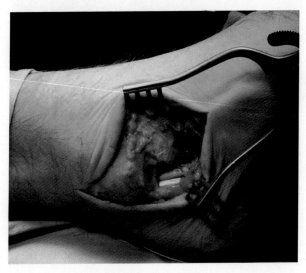

Fig. 61.3 ATFL rupture

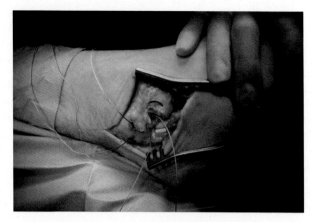

Fig. 61.4 Ankle ligament repair using suture anchors

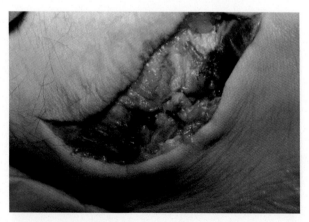

Fig. 61.5 Gould modification of Bröstrom repair

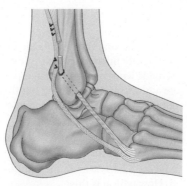

Fig. 61.6 Evans' procedure: part or all of the peroneus brevis tendon is detached proximally and threaded through the fibula

4. Following surgery, a below knee plaster is applied. This is retained either for two weeks, when it is replaced by a light ankle brace for a further 6 weeks, or simply retained with progressive weight-bearing for six weeks in total. Patients are generally able to return to most activities including light sport within a further 6 weeks.

Key Points

- Chronic ankle instability may lead to early onset joint arthritis.
- Stress radiography is useful in diagnosis
- If conservative therapy provides inadequate joint control, then surgery should be considered. A 'modified' Bröstrom anatomic repair generally provides a satisfactory result.

Further reading

Baumhauer JF, O'Brien T (2002) Surgical considerations in the treatment of ankle instability. Journal of Athletic Training 37:458–62.

Bahr R, Pena F, Shine J et al. (1997) Biomechanics of ankle ligament reconstruction. The American Journal of Sports Medicine 25:424–32.

Bröstrom L (1966) Sprained ankles. Acta Chirugica Scandinavica 132:551–65.

Kumar V, Triantafyllopoulos I, Panagopoulos A, Fitzgerald S, van Niekerk L (2007) Deficiencies of MRI in the diagnosis of chronic symptomatic lateral ankle ligament injuries. Foot and Ankle Surgery 13:171–6.

Case 62

This 45-year-old male marathon runner is plagued with pain in his right heel that intermittently interferes with his intensive training programme. Pain is made worse with running, especially uphill. His 'ankle' feels sore and stiff in the morning but this lessens after a few minutes walking. Examination reveals a tender, fusiform swelling behind his right heel (Fig. 62.1).

1. This patient has been told that he has a tenosynovitis of the Achilles tendon. Why is this incorrect?
2. The swelling in Figure 62.1 is seen in the midportion of the Achilles tendon. How typical is this?
3. What is the role of ultrasonography in diagnosing this condition?
4. What advice would you offer this patient?
5. Discuss the conservative and operative management.

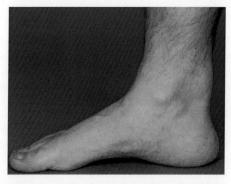

Fig. 62.1 Lateral view of heel showing a fusiform swelling in Achilles tendon

Achilles tendinopathy

1. The Achilles tendon is the largest and strongest tendon in the body. It is formed by the union of the gastrocnemius and soleus muscle tendons and inserts on the posterior aspect of the calcaneus. The Achilles tendon is covered by a thin membrane called the paratenon. It does not have a true synovial sheath and therefore 'synovitis' is a poor description.

   Ageing and high-velocity sport predispose the tendon to injury. Typically tendinopathy occurs from overuse that places abnormal biomechanical stress on the foot and ankle. The preferred, contemporary term for tendon pain, swelling and impaired performance is *tendinopathy* which encompasses and supersedes the terms tendinitis and tendinosis. Traditionally it was supposed that the pain in the tendon was due to inflammation (tendinitis) but there seems to be little evidence of this and tendons which exhibit degeneration (tendinosis) are sometimes painless. Pain with this condition may be due to neovascularization irritating pain receptors.

2. Achilles tendinopathy occurs in between 7% and 9% of top-level runners. Two-thirds of recreational athletes with Achilles tendon problems have pain in the tendon (typically 2–6 cm above insertion of tendon), as seen with this man. About 23% have insertional Achilles tendon problems and 8% have pain at the myotendinous junction. In chronic Achilles tendinopathy, peritendinous swelling often develops as shown in Figure 62.1. In such cases, about 20% of the peritendinous tissue is composed of myofibroblasts which are believed to be responsible for the formation of permanent scarring around the tendon that in turn impedes circulation.

3. Ultrasonography shows discontinuity of tendon fibres and tendon thickening. Scanning also identifies neovascularization that was once thought to signify healing but paradoxically, loose granulation tissue emerges and this leads to scarring.

4. This patient should be advised that symptoms often persist for many weeks or even months. He should be advised to reduce the intensity of his activities and to warm up thoroughly

in advance of running. This should be accompanied with advice to avoid walking barefoot or in flat-soled shoes such as slippers or sandals (it may be necessary to provide the patient with heel lifts).

5. In the early stages, oral non-steroidal anti-inflammatory drugs or topical gels and rest with ice and elevation are recommended. The patient should be given eccentric calf-stretching exercises. Control of biomechanical factors should be addressed with antipronatory orthoses. In recalcitrant cases, the use of dorsiflexion night splints or 'Strasbourg socks' should be considered although patient compliance may be an issue with these (Fig. 62.2). Because of the inherent risk of tendon rupture, steroid injections are not advocated as a routine treatment although when tendon pain does not allow eccentric stretching, a small amount of steroid, injected either side of the tendon (peritendinous), may help. Patients abstain from activity with immobilization of the ankle in a moon boot (see Fig. 56.2) or similar device.

The objective of surgery is to excise fibrotic adhesions, remove degenerated nodules and make multiple longitudinal incisions in the tendon. Risks of surgery include poor wound healing and tender scars.

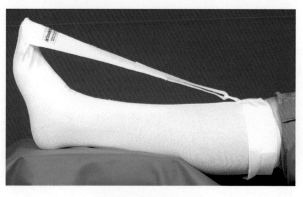

Fig. 62.2 Strasbourg sock

Evidence

In a Cochrane systematic review, three trials showed a modest benefit of NSAIDs for the alleviation of acute symptoms. There was some weak evidence of no difference compared with no treatment of low-dose heparin, heel pads, topical laser therapy and peritendinous steroid injection.

Key points

- Ageing and high-velocity sport predispose to Achilles tendinopathy.
- Typically, pain and swelling occur 2–6 cm above the insertion of tendon to the calcaneus.
- Ultrasonography is useful in diagnosing the condition and excluding tendon tear.
- Patients are given advice regarding stretching and footwear.
- Control of biomechanical factors should be addressed with antipronatory orthoses.
- Steroid injections should only be used with caution.
- Surgery removes degenerative nodules.

Further reading

Khan KM, Cook JL, Kannus P, Maffulli N, Bonar SF (2002) Time to abandon the "tendinitis" myth (editorial). British Medical Journal 324:626–7.

Maffulli N, Kader D (2002) Tendinopathy of tendo achillis. Journal of Bone and Joint Surgery 84:1–8.

McLauchlan GJ, Handoll HHG (2001) Interventions for treating acute and chronic Achilles tendinitis. Cochrane Database of Systematic Reviews, Issue 2.

Paavola M, Järvinen T, Järvinen M (2002) Achilles tendinopathy. Journal of Bone and Joint Surgery 84-A:2062–76.

Case 63

Abnormal foot mechanics have an influence on the function of the entire lower limb. A 55-year-old male dentist has recently taken up running to keep fit. He runs 4 miles three or four times per week. He would like to increase his running distance but is prevented from doing so because he suffers from pain in both shins. His pain is in the lower third of the inside of his legs. He is noted to have bilateral tibia varum (Fig. 63.1) and pronated feet on standing. The lateral borders of his shoes show excessive wear (Fig. 63.2). A fellow runner has informed him that his problem is 'shin splints' and that he requires 'orthotics'.

1. Is the fellow runner correct in his diagnosis?
2. Discuss the possible causes of this patient's pain.
3. What is the association between tibia varum and development of shin splints?
4. Will 'orthotics' help this patient?

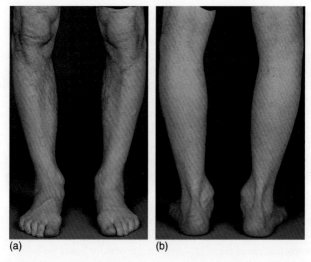

Fig. 63.1 Male runner with tibia varum and pronated feet. (a) Frontal. (b) Posterior.

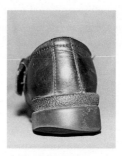

Fig. 63.2 Heel of left shoe showing excessive lateral wear

Shin splints

1. 'Shin splints' is a term used by athletes that encompasses a variety of causes of pain in the leg including soft tissue injuries, periostitis, compartment syndrome and stress fractures. In this sense, the fellow runner is correct in his assessment. However, the precise location and nature of the pain have to be determined before therapy can be applied. Shin splints may affect the anterior, lateral and posteromedial compartments of the leg.

2. The possible causes are as follows.

   Periostitis. Periostitis of the muscle attachment of tibialis posterior is due to excessive foot pronation. Tibialis posterior acts mainly to decelerate pronation and also to re-establish supination of the subtalar joint towards the end of the midstance phase of gait. Prolonged or excessive subtalar joint pronation will create a strain on the attachment of tibialis posterior to the tibia.

   Stress fracture of the tibia. Abnormal repetitive loads on bone, in this case tibia varum, mean that available pronation is used to make the foot plantigrade and therefore it loses shock absorption. Patients present with localized pain, swelling and inflammation. Suspected fractures are confirmed by radiography. Treatment is normally a short period of rest and avoidance of exercise before a gradual return to activity.

   Compartment syndrome. Exercise-induced compartment syndrome results from an increase in muscle bulk within tight fascial compartments, causing ischaemia of the enclosed muscles and nerves. Athletes present with aching or cramping in the leg as exercise progresses. Symptoms become progressively more severe and paraesthesia may be experienced in the posterior tibial nerve distribution.

3. Symptoms are related to the patient's tibia varum, because the varus alignment of the leg and foot requires compensatory subtalar joint pronation in order to make the foot plantigrade.

4. The use of an orthosis is dependent on the cause. This patient was diagnosed as having a periostitis of the tibia at the attachment of tibialis posterior muscle and therefore an orthosis was successful in limiting foot pronation. Figure 63.3 shows a custom-made orthosis consisting of a medial heel wedge designed to reduce abnormal foot pronation.

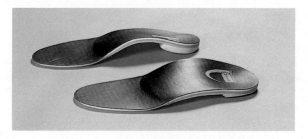

Fig. 63.3 In-shoe orthoses with a medial heel wedge

Key points

- Shin splints are an overuse injury of the leg.
- They may occur as a result of excessive subtalar joint pronation.
- Orthoses improve symptoms when the cause is a soft tissue injury.
- Other causes of shin splints are stress fracture of the tibia and compartment syndrome.

Further reading

Rzonca EC, Baylis WJ (1988) Common sports injuries to the foot and leg. Clinics in Podiatric Medicine and Surgery 5(3):591–611.

Subotnick SI (1975) Shin splint syndrome of the lower extremity. In: Podiatric Sports Medicine. New York: Futura Publishing Company, 79–81.

Case 64

A soccer player presents to A&E having injured his right foot during a tackle when his foot was forced into inversion. He was aware of an audible crack. On examination, the dorsum of the left forefoot is inflamed, swollen and extremely tender. A radiograph is requested (Fig. 64.1).

1. Which eponym is associated with fracture of the base of the fifth metatarsal?
2. Describe the three recognized types of fifth metatarsal shaft fractures.
3. Which of these fractures is most challenging to treat and why?
4. Discuss the management of these fractures.
5. A number of high-profile sportsmen (including Wayne Rooney and Michael Owen) have recently suffered from such a fracture. Why is this?

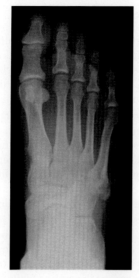

Fig. 64.1 AP radiograph of foot

Fractures of the proximal fifth metatarsal

1. In 1902 Sir Robert Jones wrote an article entitled 'Fracture of the base of the fifth metatarsal bone by indirect violence'. The injury was reported in six patients, one of whom was himself. He had sustained the injury while Maypole dancing. The article included a description of fractures in three zones.

2. Figure 64.2 illustrates the zones. Avulsion fractures of the fifth metatarsal arise in zone 1 after the peroneus brevis muscle tendon is tightened by forced inversion of the foot as was shown in Figure 64.1. A fragment of bone separates from the bone along the apophyseal line of the fifth metatarsal base. This fracture should be differentiated from os vesalianum and the apophysitis of the fifth metatarsal (Iselin's disease).

   Jones' fractures occur in zone 2 (zone of Jones' fracture) (Fig. 64.3), at the junction of the shaft and base, at the level of the distal limit of the joint between the fourth and fifth metatarsals. They are the result of a sudden thrust of the lateral border of the foot against the ground while the heel is raised.

   Stress fractures (or fatigue fractures) occur in the proximal 1.5 cm of the diaphysis (Fig. 64.4; Zone 3).

3. Jones' fractures can be challenging to treat because they are prone to delayed or non-union. This is thought to be caused by vascular insufficiency as the nutrient artery to the base of the bone enters medially at midshaft level and passes proximally.

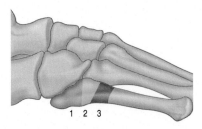

Fig. 64.2 Illustration of three fracture zones in the proximal fifth metatarsal

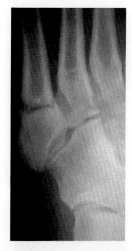

Fig. 64.3 Zone 2: Jones' fracture

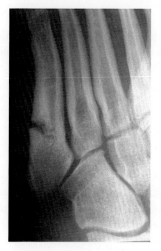

Fig. 64.4 Zone 3: stress fracture

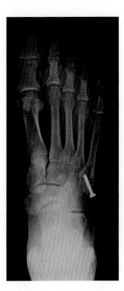

Fig. 64.5 Internal fixation of fracture

4. Avulsion and stress fractures generally heal if the foot is immobilized in a cast for 4–6 weeks. Jones' fractures require stabilization as shown in Figure 64.5.
5. Lighter, less supportive boots are blamed for an increase in foot fractures in footballers. There is also a tendency for footballers to wear boots which are too tight and this might compound the problem.

Key points

- There are three types of fracture of the fifth metatarsal base.
- Up to 50% non-union rate reported after 2 months.
- Stabilization of Jones' fracture is recommended.

Further reading

Fetzer GB, Wright RW (2006) Metatarsal shaft fractures and fractures of the proximal fifth metatarsal. Clinics in Sports Medicine 25(1):139–50.

Jones R (1902) Fracture of the fifth metatarsal bone by indirect violence. Annals of Surgery 35:697–700.

Petrisor BA, Ekrol I, Court-Brown C (2006) The epidemiology of metatarsal fractures. Foot and Ankle International 27(3):172–4.

Torg JS, Balduini FC, Zelko RR, Pavlov H, Peff TC, Das M (1984) Fracture of the base of the fifth metatarsal distal to the tuberosity. Classification and guidelines for non-surgical and surgical management. Journal of Bone and Joint Surgery 66-A:209–14.

Case 65

Sesamoid bones can be the source of pathology. This 29-year-old schoolteacher was playing tennis in September. She described jumping for a smash, landing heavily and immediately feeling pain in her big toe joint. It is now February and her pain has not improved. It is worse on walking and relieved by rest. Examination reveals a high-arched foot, a plantarflexed first ray and tenderness in the region of her medial sesamoid bone. Radiographs of her first MTP joint and sesamoids are as shown (Fig. 65.1).

1. Has this tennis player fractured her sesamoid bone or is this a bipartite sesamoid? Which is more likely?
2. What other conditions affect the sesamoids?
3. What is the treatment for sesamoid pain?
4. When is surgery of the sesamoid bones considered?

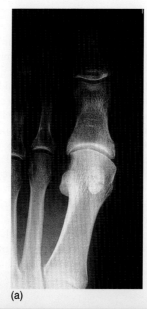

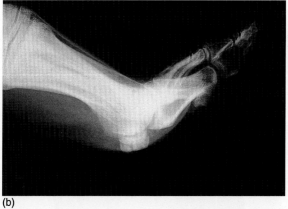

Fig. 65.1 (a) AP radiographs. (b) Lateral radiographs of sesamoid bones

Sesamoiditis

1. True fracture of the sesamoids is rare and fractures are more likely to be stress related. Fractures should be differentiated from partite sesamoids, which are commonplace, occurring in approximately 25% of individuals. In 80% the medial sesamoid is affected and 90% of the total are bilateral. A fractured sesamoid is not corticated at its fracture line and is only slightly longer than its normal neighbours. A bipartite or tripartite sesamoid is usually larger than a single sesamoid and the partite segments are oval with smooth concave/convex opposing edges (Fig. 65.2). Although partite sesamoids are much more common, given the history, this patient's symptoms and the radiological appearances, it would appear that she does have a fracture of her medial sesamoid.

2. Sesamoid bones can be affected by the same spectrum of pathology as any other bone. Sesamoiditis (chondromalacia) may occur from repetitive mechanical stress, osteochondritis

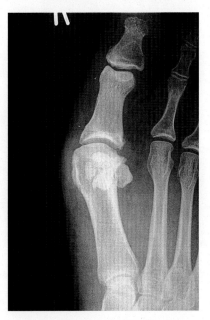

Fig. 65.2 Tripartite medial sesamoid bone

from injury (characterized by mottling of the sesamoid on X-ray), degenerative arthritis, inflammatory arthritis and infection.

3. Regardless of cause, the first-line treatment for sesamoid pain is to offload pressure from the first MTP joint and the sesamoids. In most instances, an insole with a plantar metatarsal pad achieves this by deflecting pressure from the first metatarsal head. In the event of non-union of a fractured sesamoid, immobilization in a cast may be indicated. In-shoe plantar pressure measurements provide a useful means of evaluating the effectiveness of orthoses by quantifying pressure reduction (Fig. 65.3). In this case, these simple measures were sufficient to significantly ameliorate the patient's symptoms. Figure 65.3a shows maximum pressures 54 Ncm^{-2} and 40 Ncm^{-2} under the right and left metatarsal heads respectively. Figure 65.3b shows the same feet, this time with an insole in the right shoe. Pressure at the metatarsal head has been reduced to 16 Ncm^{-2} on the right side, while on the left the pressure remains high.

4. Surgical excision of part or all of one sesamoid may be considered for non-union of a fractured bone or avascular necrosis. It should be explained to the patient that relief of pain is not guaranteed. The flexor digitorum brevis tendon must be kept intact to prevent an extension deformity of the hallux.

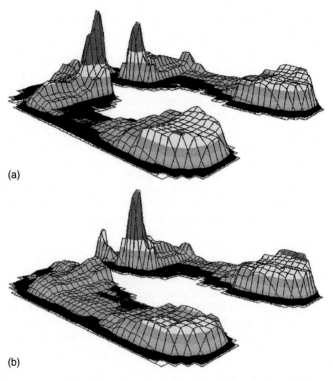

(a)

(b)

Fig. 65.3 In-shoe right foot pressures, (a) without insole and (b) with insole

Clinical tip: plantar pressure assessment

Plantar pressures give a good indication of foot function during gait, by quantitatively measuring the distribution of load under the foot. The example above illustrates the use of the Novel™ Pedar system. This system utilizes insoles placed within the patient's shoes. The measurement of pressures at the foot–shoe interface is the one that most resembles 'real-life' walking and it also allows the analysis of a number of steps and other activities. However, the nature of the flexible insole compromises reliability compared to fixed-force platforms which provide a true vertical force measurement. Force platforms also contain more sensors, and therefore have greater resolution of data, but they suffer from the need for patients to 'target' the platform, which may alter normal gait.

With improving technology, measurement of plantar pressure is becoming more commonplace in the clinical environment. Measurements are invaluable for the assessment of patients regarded as being at risk from high plantar pressures, particularly with diabetes and rheumatoid arthritis. Once the patient is identified as having abnormal plantar pressures, the efficacy of various therapies such as footwear, orthoses and surgery can be evaluated, as in the case example above.

Key points

- True fractures of the hallux sesamoid bones are rare; they are usually stress related.
- Fracture should be differentiated from partite sesamoids.
- Sesamoid pain is treated with deflective insoles.
- Plantar foot pressure assessment is useful in assessing the effectiveness of insoles.

Further reading

Munuera PV, Domínguez G, Reina M, Trujillo P (2007) Bipartite hallucal sesamoid bones: relationship with hallux valgus and metatarsal index. Skeletal Radiology 36(11):1043–50.

Orlin MN, McPoil TG (2000) Plantar pressure assessment. Physical Therapy 80:399–409.

Richardson E (1987) Injuries to the hallucal sesamoid in the athlete. Foot and Ankle International 7:229–44.

Rosenfield JS, Trepman E (2000) Treatment of sesamoid disorders with a rocker sole shoe modification. Foot and Ankle International 21(4):914–15.

Scranton P, Rutkowski R (1980) Anatomic variations in the first ray. Part II. Disorders of the sesamoids. Clinical Orthopaedics and Related Research 151:256–64.

Section 10

Multiple choice questions

Select the single best answer for each question:

1. With regard to injuries at the Lisfranc joint, which of the following is true?
   A. Arthrodesis is indicated for primarily ligamentous injuries
   B. Lisfranc's ligament tethers the first and second metatarsal bases
   C. The navicular is dislocated
   D. The severity of the injury is less important than the final position
   E. The third metatarsal is the keystone

2. Which of the following is NOT a feature of Marfan's syndrome?
   A. Aortic arch anomalies
   B. Brachydactyly
   C. Dislocation of the lens
   D. High arched palate
   E. Scoliosis

3. After a bite by a pit viper which of the following is most appropriate?
   A. Antivenom in the field
   B. Application of pressure immobilization
   C. Apply ice to the limb
   D. Electroshock therapy
   E. Sucking the wound

4. A middle-aged lady presents with left pes planovalgus. Examination reveals that she is unable to rise onto her toes on that side. After correction of her heel into neutral the forefoot remains rigidly supinated. Which would you treat her by?
   A. Pan-talar arthrodesis
   B. Tendon transfer and calcaneal osteotomy
   C. Tendon transfer, calcaneal osteotomy and medical cuneiform osteotomy
   D. Tenosynovectomy of tibialis posterior tendon
   E. Triple arthrodesis

5. A 20 year old suffers a Hawkins type III fracture of the talus. Which of the following is true?
    A. Regardless of the surgical treatment of this fracture, weight bearing should be delayed for 18 months to allow the talus to revascularize
    B. The subtalar joint is subluxed but the ankle joint normal
    C. There is a 90% rate of avascular necrosis of the body of the talus after this fracture
    D. There is a 90% rate of non-union of this fracture
    E. Those fractures treated conservatively tend to go into valgus

6. Which of the following is true with respect to calcaneal fracture?
    A. Approximately 60% are sustained in a fall from a height
    B. Böhler's angle is increased to greater than 40°
    C. Greater than 50% of fractures are extra-articular in adults
    D. Reduced triceps surae power is a serious clinical problem
    E. Sustentaculum fracture rarely occurs as an isolated fracture

7. In poliomyelitis:
    A. Classically patients develop an equinovarus foot
    B. Feet affected by polio may be cold and blue
    C. Full leg braces are seldom required
    D. Heel varus is associated with forefoot valgus
    E. Muscle wasting only affects the foot extensors

8. In the treatment of an acute attack of gout:
    A. Prescribe allopurinol, building the dose up to 300 mg/day
    B. Prescribe colchicine in increasing dosage if renal function impaired
    C. Prescribe indomethacin and start allopurinol at high dose
    D. Prescribe probenecid and increase fluid intake
    E. Prescribe probenecid and reduce fluid intake

9. **Regarding cartilaginous tumours in the foot:**
   A. Chondrosarcomas are generally multiple
   B. Deep endosteal scalloping is characteristic of an enchondroma
   C. Lesions in the hindfoot are more likely to be malignant than those in the forefoot
   D. Malignant transformation from enchondroma is common
   E. The lesions are generally entirely radiolucent

10. **A patient presents with a discolouration under her second toe nail. Would you?**
   A. Amputate the digit immediately
   B. Arrange admission for excisional biopsy
   C. Assume that as there is no lymphadenopathy the lesion is benign
   D. Note with interest and arrange to review in 3 months
   E. Wedge resect the nail and shave the lesion

11. **A child presents with metatarsus adductus.**
   A. It is the most common cause of intoeing gait in children with diplegic cerebral palsy
   B. It will increase the first-second intermetatarsal angle (IMA) in patients with hallux valgus
   C. Long-term deformity is generally to be expected
   D. Split lateral anterior tibialis tendon transfer may be required to address muscle imbalance
   E. The majority of patients require surgical intervention

12. **A 3-year-old presents with congenital curling of her third toe. Treatment should consist of:**
   A. A Girdlestone flexor digitorum longus to extensor digitorum transfer
   B. Excision of the PIP joint of the toe
   C. Lengthening of the extensor digitorum tendon and release of the dorsal joint capsule
   D. Stretching exercises and taping up of the digit
   E. Tenotomy of the flexor digitorum longus and brevis to the toe

13. **In paediatric flat foot:**
    A. Flattening of the talar axis to metatarsal base angle is characteristic
    B. Peroneal muscular atrophy is associated
    C. Peroneal spasticity is associated
    D. Sport should be restricted to prevent worsening of the condition
    E. Supports should be prescribed in infancy

14. **In clubfoot:**
    A. Calf wasting is only evident in childhood
    B. The condition is more common in females
    C. The condition is rarely bilateral
    D. There is a greater than 20% risk in subsequent offspring
    E. Turco's angle is >35°

15. **In venous insufficiency which of the following is FALSE?**
    A. Doppler scanning is required
    B. Leg elevation helps to reduce hydrostatic pressure
    C. Melanin causes extensive discolouration in the 'gaiter' region of the legs
    D. Stanozol may be used in ulcer management
    E. Varicosities arise from incompetence of the supercial venous valves

16. **With respect to plantar fibromatosis:**
    A. Collagenase injection into Dupuytren tissue is ineffective
    B. It commonly causes toe flexion contractures
    C. Plantar fibroma commonly invade the skin
    D. Palmar-plantar fibromatosis may occur in children less than 12 years old
    E. Radiotherapy will reduce symptoms but does not influence disease progression

17. **In forefoot metatarsalgia:**
    A. A Keller's arthroplasty will shorten the great toe metatarsal
    B. Callosity resection by excision of an ellipse of plantar skin may be adequate

C. The forefoot fat pad lies distal to the metatarsal heads

D. The primary problem is a weakness of the toe flexor muscles

E. Weil's osteotomy is designed to displace the metatarsal heads dorsally

18. A 32-year-old footballer has grade 2 hallux rigidus. What would your favoured treatment be?
    A. Dorsal cheilectomy
    B. Fusion of the metatarsophalangeal joint
    C. Keller's resection arthroplasty
    D. Mojé ceramic toe replacement
    E. Swanson silastic arthroplasty

19. Which of the following conditions is NOT a cause of macrodactyly?
    A. Arteriovenous fistula
    B. Macrodystrophia lipomatosa
    C. Marfan's syndrome
    D. Multiple enchondromatosis
    E. Neurofibromatosis

20. With regard to hallux limitus/rigidus, which of the following is true?
    A. First-ray hypermobility is a functional variation that results in degeneration of the first MTP joint
    B. Hallux flexus is the cause of hallux limitus
    C. Normal dorsiflexion at the first MTP joint is $<30°$
    D. Patients have a high serum urate
    E. The use of intra-articular steroid injections is not supported

21. Regarding Freiberg's infraction, which of the following statements is true?
    A. Freiberg's infraction only occurs in adolescents
    B. Gauthier's procedure involves rotating the dorsal cartilage onto the articulating surface

C. 'Infraction' describes collapse of the metatarsal head
D. In stage I of the Smillie classification, bone absorption has taken place
E. Joint replacement is not indicated for Freiberg's

22. **In respect of plantar fasciitis:**
   A. heel spurs are present in >90%
   B. pain is worse in the evening
   C. the condition is self-limiting
   D. the evidence base supports the use of extracorporeal shockwave therapy
   E. X-rays are required for definitive diagnosis

23. **Which of the following is the most useful treatment for Haglund's bump?**
   A. Heel lifts
   B. Injection of steroid
   C. Non-steroidal anti-inflammatory medication
   D. Non-weightbearing casts
   E. Soft pads to protect posterior prominence

24. **With regard to ganglia, which of the following statements is true?**
   A. Aspiration of ganglia followed by corticosteroid injection is risk free
   B. Ganglia greater than 2 cm in diameter must be excised
   C. Multiple ganglia are present in neurofibromatosis
   D. They are fluid-filled cystic swellings that transilluminate
   E. They contain mucus

25. **With regard to plantar pustulosis/dermatosis, which of the following is true?**
   A. It may be spread by hand contact
   B. Juvenile plantar dermatosis is a contact dermatitis caused by detergents
   C. Palmoplantar pustulosis is a localized form of psoriasis
   D. Steroid creams should be avoided
   E. The condition is of fungal origin

26. With regard to fungal infections of the toenails, which of the following is true?
    A. Griseofulvin is the mainstay of treatment
    B. The condition is more common in younger people
    C. There are four genera of dermatophytes that infect the nail
    D. Topical treatments are not effective in treating the toenail
    E. Treatment is not always required

27. With regard to ingrowing toenails, which of the following is true?
    A. Antibiotics effectively resolve the problem
    B. Incurvature of the toenail is also referred to as 'onychocryptosis'
    C. Phenol is a strong alkali
    D. Phenolization is not always recommended after removal of toenail
    E. There is a high risk of regrowth following Zadik's or Winograd's procedures alone

28. With regard to subungual exostosis, which of the following is true?
    A. A solitary exostosis is rare
    B. It arises from the nail matrix
    C. It is an osteochondroma
    D. They occur more commonly in the foot than the hand
    E. They occur primarily in elderly patients

29. With regard to plantar warts, which statement is true?
    A. Duct tape is effective in the treatment of warts because of the allergic reaction to the adhesive
    B. Human papilloma virus is associated with epithelial overgrowth
    C. Mosaic warts are only seen in immunosuppressed individuals
    D. Viral material affects the basal layer of the epidermis
    E. Warts do not resolve spontaneously

30. **With regard to pitted keratolysis, which statement is true?**
    A. Human papilloma virus is isolated from skin scrapings
    B. The condition is best treated with emollients
    C. There is a fungal infection of the skin
    D. There is an overgrowth of *Cornyebacterium diphtheriae*
    E. Topical antibiotics are ineffective

31. **Which of the following statements is true of talocalcaneal synostosis?**
    A. Bar excision can be considered at any time
    B. MR scans are required routinely
    C. Talar beaking is pathognomonic
    D. Tip toe standing is not possible
    E. X-rays utilizing Harris views confirm diagnosis

32. **Which of the following constitutes the triad of Reiter's syndrome?**
    A. Arthritis, urethritis and pitting of the nails
    B. Balanitis, conjunctivitis and spondylitis
    C. Conjunctivitis, urethritis and arthritis
    D. Keratoderma blennorrhagicum, spondylitis and conjunctivitis
    E. Plantar fasciitis, urethritis and keratoderma blennorrhagicum

33. **Which of the following set of symptoms is most strongly indicative of Morton's neuroma?**
    A. Dorsal swelling
    B. Numbness in the third and fourth toes
    C. Pain in the forefoot regardless of the style of shoes
    D. Pain in the third and fourth toes immediately on weightbearing
    E. Pain in the toes at night

34. **Which of the following statements about diabetic neuropathy is false?**
    A. Autonomic neuropathy causes increased hydration of the skin
    B. Autonomic neuropathy leads to arteriovenous shunting

C. Clawing of the toes is evidence of motor neuropathy

D. Sensory loss occurs in a 'glove and stocking' distribution

E. Sensory neuropathy can be tested with a 10g Semmes-Weinstein monofilament

35. **Which of the following is not a cause of vitiligo?**

A. Addison's hypoadrenalism

B. Diabetes

C. Hashimoto's thyroiditis

D. Pernicious anaemia

E. Rheumatoid arthritis

36. **In the treatment of Achilles tendinopathy, steroid injections:**

A. Allow early return to activities

B. Break down nodular swelling

C. Must always be injected with local anaesthetic

D. Risk rupture of the tendon

E. Stimulate nociceptors

37. **Pigmented vilonodular synovitis:**

A. Calcification is a usual feature of the PVNS lesion

B. Causes painless joint/tendon sheath swelling

C. Is characterized by haemosiderin-laden multinucleate giant cells

D. Rarely results in bone cyst formation

E. Spreads through draining lymphatics

38. **Which of the following is true of metatarsal stress fracture?**

A. Fractures are not apparent until endosteal or periosteal bone callus becomes evident

B. It is caused by normal forces applied to abnormal bone

C. Non-union necessitates open reduction and internal fixation

D. Radio-isotope bone scans (scintigraphs) utilizing technetium phosphate 99mTc (half-life 6 hours) detects metabolic bone changes within 2 weeks

E. The incidence is greater in spring time

MCQ Answers

1. Answer A
2. Answer B
3. Answer B
4. Answer C
5. Answer C
6. Answer E
7. Answer B
8. Answer B
9. Answer C
10. Answer B
11. Answer D
12. Answer E
13. Answer C
14. Answer D
15. Answer E
16. Answer D
17. Answer C
18. Answer A
19. Answer C
20. Answer A
21. Answer C
22. Answer C
23. Answer E
24. Answer D
25. Answer C
26. Answer E
27. Answer E
28. Answer D
29. Answer B
30. Answer D
31. Answer C
32. Answer C
33. Answer B
34. Answer A
35. Answer E
36. Answer D
37. Answer C
38. Answer A

CASE LIST

Section 1 Paediatrics

1. Congenital talipes equinovarus
2. Accessory navicular
3. Flat foot
4. Claw toe and adductus quinti digiti
5. Kohler's disease
6. Metatarsus adductus
7. Talocalcaneal synostosis
8. Congenital metatarsal anomalies

Section 2 Lumps and bumps

9. Tarsometatarsal arthritis (tarsal boss)
10. Ganglion
11. Neurothekeoma (nerve sheath myxoma)
12. Plantar fibroma
13. Subungual exostosis

Section 3 Orthopaedics

14. Aetiology of hallux rigidus
15. Freiberg's infraction
16. Hammer toe
17. Polydactyly and macrodactyly
18. Aetiology of hallux valgus
19. Plantar fasciitis
20. Haglund's syndrome
21. Surgery of hallux rigidus
22. Metatarsalgia
23. Surgery of hallux valgus

Section 4 Dermatology

24. Vitiligo
25. Venous ulceration
26. Plantar pustulosis/dermatosis
27. Fungal foot infections
28. Ingrowing toenails
29. Plantar warts
30. Pitted keratolysis
31. Chilblains with Raynaud's phenomenon

Section 5 At-risk foot

32. Septic arthritis
33. Critical limb ischaemia
34. Snake bite
35. Melanoma
36. Amputation
37. Ischaemic toe
38. Chondrosarcoma of the great toe
39. Frostbite
40. Subcutaneous infection
41. Pressure sores

Section 6 Rheumatology

42. Benign joint hypermobility syndrome
43. Diagnosis of rheumatoid arthritis
44. Pigmented villonodular synovitis/giant cell tumour of tendon sheath
45. Gout
46. Reiter's syndrome
47. Psoriatic arthritis
48. Therapy of rheumatoid arthritis

Section 7 Neurology

Section 8 Trauma

Section 9 Sports injuries

Section 10 Multiple choice questions

Index

Printed in the United States
By Bookmasters